HOW TO MAKE LOVE TO A YOUNGER MAN

HOW TO MAKE LOVE TO A YOUNGER MAN

ILONA PARIS

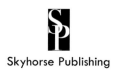

Skyhorse Publishing

Skyhorse Publishing books may be purchased in bulk at special discounts for sales promotion, corporate gifts, fund-raising, or educational purposes. Special editions can also be created to specifications. For details, contact the Special Sales Department, Skyhorse Publishing, 307 West 36th Street, 11th Floor, New York, NY 10018 or info@skyhorsepublishing.com.

Skyhorse® and Skyhorse Publishing® are registered trademarks of Skyhorse Publishing, Inc.®, a Delaware corporation.

Visit our website at www.skyhorsepublishing.com.

10 9 8 7 6 5 4 3 2

Paperback ISBN: 978-1-62636-030-3

Library of Congress Cataloging-in-Publication Data

Paris, Ilona.
    Hot cougar sex : steamy encounters with younger men / Ilona Paris.
        p. cm.
    ISBN 978-1-60239-348-6 (alk. paper)
    1. Middle-aged women—Sexual behavior. 2. Middle-aged women—Attitudes. 3. Young men—Sexual behavior. 4. Sex. 5. Man-woman relationships. I. Title.
    HQ29.P37 2008
    306.77084'4—dc22
                                                                2008027152

Printed in China

CONTENTS

Introduction

Tasting the Young Delectable: An Urban Delight

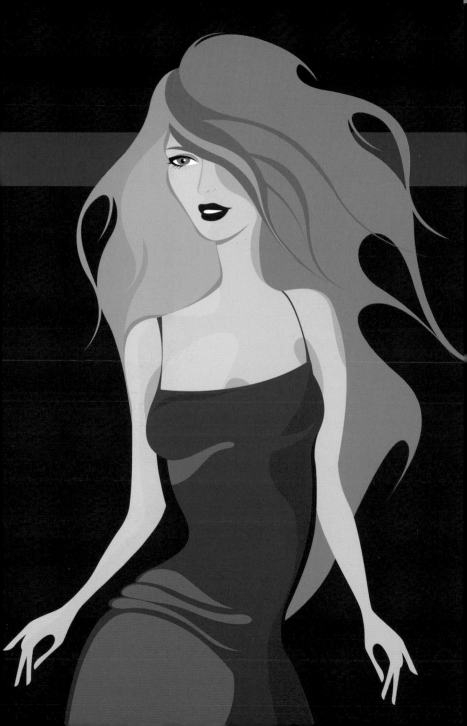

Well, it was bound to happen sooner or later. One day I started to develop a penchant for young men. I found myself gaping at photos of Calvin Klein models, those washboard abs, the V shape of their hips right before the top of their jeans, those sweeping shoulders, and the flesh—that tight, hot, smooth flesh. I found myself almost driving off the road when I saw a shirtless young college student jogging down the street. God help me, the yearning within me was a surprise and somewhat of an embarrassment.

It was at this time that I learned that the Urban Cougar is a sophisticated species of female who takes her pleasure from a younger male. She is a feline who prefers the freedom of the hunt as opposed to being tied down to a relationship. She has shaken the taboos that our society has tried to dictate and is true to herself and her desires. She loves adventure and isn't afraid to let her hair down and go after what she wants.

In our society, for a woman who has entered her forties, it is as if life is suddenly over. This just doesn't seem right to me. Why is it acceptable for an older man to go out with a younger woman, but not for an older woman to go out with a younger man? The glorification of marriage and motherhood has been the banner flying across our city streets since the '50s. I say, "Ahh, bullshit."

Women today are stunning, with great careers and education. We are well traveled and in great shape. We have all sorts of great things at our fingertips: Botox, plastic surgery, yoga, and health spas to help us buff our cougar bodies to a beautiful sheen. We can strut down the sidewalk in our Manolos with pride and confidence, giving young men a sniff at what we possess.

I remember sitting to attention while watching a segment of *Oprah* in which she featured women who were marrying younger men. This made sense to me. A younger man could keep up with me. I found that as I entered my second adulthood, somewhere around the age of forty, I had so much energy. A man my age, in his late fifties or early sixties, was getting ready for retirement and in a lot of cases didn't put the effort into his physical appearance that I did. A younger man did, however. Sitting in front of the TV every night with an old man simply was not on my agenda. I was going out and hitting the town.

Older woman are able to experience a new freedom; we don't have to juggle young children and family life. Activity is key to leading an exuberant life at this stage. Having lots of sex can help with this and also release endorphins, which are known to be a feel-good hormone. Sex is also an incredible beauty treatment. Look at someone who is having a great sex life and they just radiate. A woman can experience a new freedom in her sex life that can just knock her panties right off!

Demi Moore boldly went where we all wanted to go, which was to marry her boy toy, Ashton Kutcher. Ay caramba, that was hot stuff. Tina Turner, the sexy rocker, married a man twenty years her junior, and Joan Collins's husband is three decades younger than she is. Mae West, always ahead of her time, was well into her nineties with a lover forty-five years younger than she. She stated, "It is not the men in my life who count—it is the life in my men." There is clearly something to this, and things are changing. These are stunning examples of cougars who are purring loudly.

The younger guy doesn't have hang-ups like the men in our generation. He is ready for the challenge. He is forging new paths with his cougar. Some young men find older women more sophisticated. We can maintain an air of mystique that our younger selves did not. The cougar has been molded by her many life experiences, and as a result has substance. A young man can jump-start a women's self-confidence, while the mature woman has the ability to boost a young man's ego. He loves the feeling that his cougar is giving him: an encounter with the ultimate in sophistication. The bonus is they have the ability to ignite a delicious new sensuality in each other.

A cougar finds that her young lover regenerates her juicy self. The Europeans have long known the allure of the femme fatale over fifty. She is worldly, with a treasure trove of erotic delights just waiting to be discovered, admired, and appreciated.

And most appealing: these days, you can rob that cradle and not feel guilty about it. A woman can overcome all the taboos related to her sexual identity and embrace her sexiness. If young hot stuff is what you want, don't be afraid of it. Embrace your animal charisma and growl in sheer delight, my friends. Feel free to prowl through the streets looking for that marvelous hot thing and pounce when you have found him. You will find it is a delightful boost to your ego. I found getting it on with a younger man put zest in my step and made my heart a bit lighter. Life is too hard not to have fun. Meow.

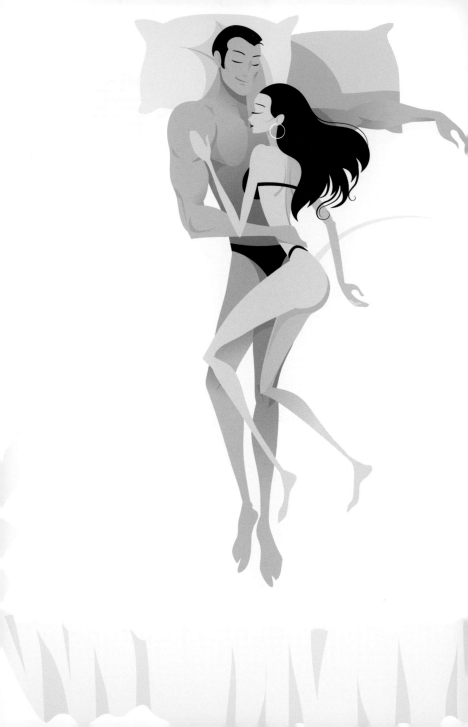

Goth Dude

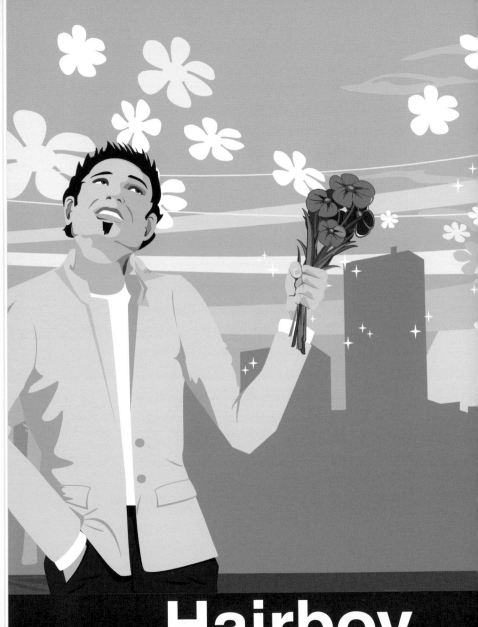

Hairboy

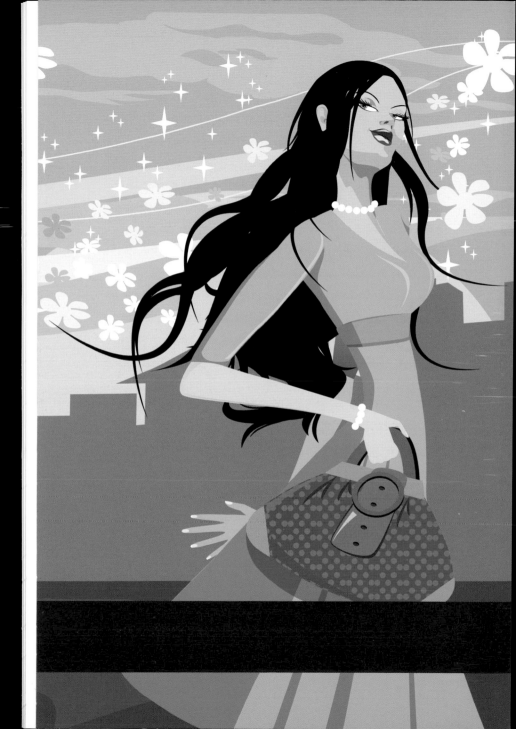

Mr. Handsome

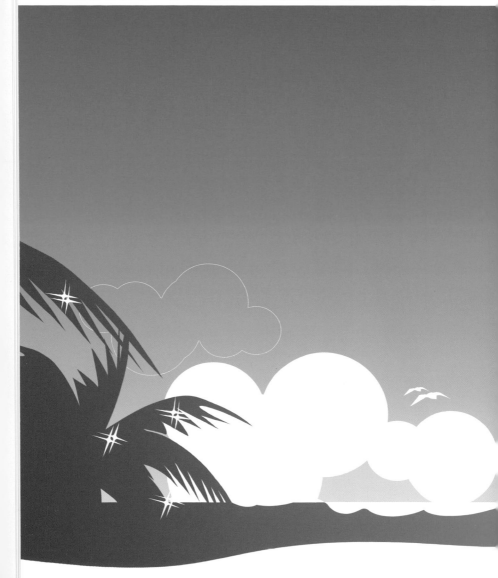

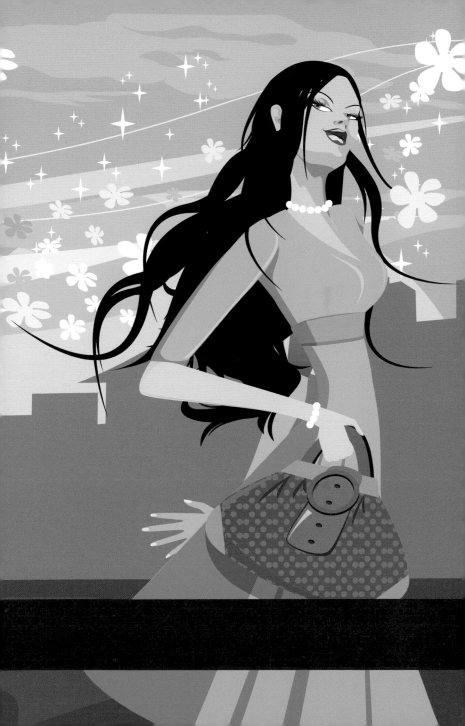

Once I had drunk from the fountain of youth, I wanted more of this divine elixir. I suddenly felt alive again. I had a spring in my step when I walked down the street. So I was thrilled when I didn't have to wait long for my next escapade. A young man came into my office one day, and I immediately sat up to take notice. He was twenty-eight (my favorite number), 6'2", with spiked hair that stuck up and out like that of a rock star. He was dressed in a violet shirt, sleek black pants, and giant black sunglasses. He had silver rings on his fingers and a heavy matching chain around his neck. It was all I could do not to jump over the front desk and wrap my legs around this luscious specimen.

I promptly named him Hairboy, because his hair had so much product in it to achieve this crazy look. His looks were clearly important to this young creature. Hairboy was also a health fanatic, as evidenced by his constantly drinking protein drinks. Since he was staying in Boston for a few days to work on a special project with our company, I thought I would do what any citizen might do and offer to show him our town. "Would you like to go to my health club and work out?" I asked. Of course he did, who wouldn't? I worked hard at being cougarlicious. I would pick him up at his hotel after work. I quickly ran home and put on my cutest workout outfit. I was a cougar on the prowl.

I scooped Hairboy up at his hotel and we blasted down the highway in Shirley. When we got to the health club, he looked fit to be eaten in his workout clothes. And then there were his bulging biceps. The thought of anything bulging on this guy got me quite excited. I would steal looks at this gorgeous creature wiping the sweat from his body every once in a while. Maybe I should help him. When we finished our workout it turned out Hairboy wanted to shower, but not at the club because of germs. Okay. Again, as any good citizen would, I offered my home. The writing was on the wall that this guy wanted to get naked in my home.

While he was showering I put on my finest lingerie, touched up my makeup, and brushed my hair. I must say I was having a particularly good hair day, thank God. I looked in the mirror and thought, *Damn, I look good for forty-nine.* Forty-five minutes later Hairboy was still in the shower. I poked my head in the door and asked if he was still alive. Later, when I went to use them, I would find out that he had been sampling every beauty product I possessed. The pièce de résistance was when he asked if I had any underwear he could borrow. The joys of dating a young metrosexual were just beginning to blossom for me.

"Do you want a pair of panties?" I asked.

He wanted to know if I had any men's boxers lying around. *Does this look like Bloomingdale's?* I really couldn't wait any longer. I grabbed him and slipped my hand around his waist.

"I don't think you will need any underwear, my dear," I purred.

This man was so physically gorgeous that I wanted to eat him up. Hairboy was like an art deco sculpture. His body was chiseled from working out and drinking all those protein drinks. There was something physically delicious about his skin. Kissing him was akin to savoring an umeboshi plum.

I guided him backward into my bedroom and pushed him onto my bed. My cat, Sushi, went running for the hills. She probably thought, "Not this again." This man could kiss. I was in heaven. I have found that at this stage in my life I get particularly juicy when I am kissing a pair of succulent lips. He hadn't put product in his hair, so it just kind of framed his face. The way he held his head reminded me of a wild thoroughbred horse whose neck I just wanted to stroke. I really was struck by this man's elegance.

His cock wasn't very long, but it was as strong as if he had been lifting weights with it during his workouts. Well, I was ready to put him through his paces. My passion seemed to rise from my inner core and take over my soul. I am cougar— hear me roar. I pounced above him and straddled his hips. I bent over and kissed him deeply. I lowered my hips and rubbed my seeping pussy along his shaft. It was hard between my lips. I slid up and down him, imagining sliding on a silken slope in the Alps where the air was fine. His leather-wristed hands grasped mine as he flipped me on my back. I raised my legs up around his neck and hoisted my hips to meet his cock. It slid in and felt wonderful. Up and up— those Pilates moves were coming in handy—I reached my hips to meet his. (Seriously, if you take Pilates, try to use the "C" curve with your abdomen to scoop in and out toward his cock. You will find your stamina to be amazing.) My cunt sucked him in with an intensity I couldn't stop. He started to thrust with such strength that I was surprised at the power of his cock. May I say I was a happy woman at this particular moment? Thank God we had worked out beforehand. This was Olympic fucking, my dears, and I think we both scored a ten that day.

I did not come with this person and found I really didn't need to. There is something to be said for enhanced lovemaking without orgasm. Some spiritual traditions believe withholding orgasm provides a more intense experience because you are able to make love for a much longer period of time. This was true with Hairboy. We would go at it, rest, and continue. I liked the physical stamina we both possessed, and the art of pleasing each other continued for a long time.

I must admit I became a bit winded at the end. I was conscious of this because all I could think of was, *This guy is going to think I am old and can't hack it.* It was strange to be thinking this way and I had to kick it out of my mind real quick so I didn't get weird.

We were lying on the bed and I was in his arms feeling quite comfy when Hairboy asked, "May I ask you something personal?"

"Sure," I responded.

"How old are you?"

I thought, *Oh, here we go.* "I'm forty-nine," I said.

"WHAT!" he shrieked.

At that very moment, I wanted to crawl into the ground. He just kept shouting it out loud, "Forty-nine! Forty-nine? Forty-nine!" I wasn't sure if strangulation or stabbing was in order at that moment. He then realized how traumatized I was.

He said, "It isn't an insult, I just can't believe it. I thought you were maybe thirty-five."

I couldn't speak. I just wanted him to leave. This can happen when you date someone younger. You need to be prepared for it if possible.

"I mean, I didn't think you were that old. I thought maybe you were forty," he said.

At this point I was really ready to kill him. I just wanted him to leave.

"Can't we at least talk about it?" he asked.

"You are just digging a deeper hole for yourself." I said. "I just can't talk to you right now," I continued, as I pulled on a T-shirt.

"I am really sorry," he said. "I was just so surprised.

"It is just the wrong thing to say to a woman right after you have had sex."

We were able to talk through it, but it rocked me. I

just couldn't believe the physical beauty this man possessed. He truly was scrumptious. I thought I would at least let him sit down and try to make polite conversation before I swooped down on him. We sat on the sofa and discussed his day. I asked what he had for dinner and where. I could have given a flying hoot, frankly. My pheromones must have taken effect because he reached over and placed me on his lap. *Oh, here we go.* This was working for me. Again, he possessed me with that mouth. *Mmmm.* He slipped

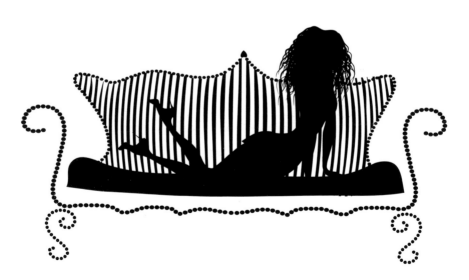

me onto the purple suede settee that was in front of the sofa and I lay back with my legs spread on either side facing him. Being a cougar, I have reached an age where I feel secure enough to wallow in my freedom. I stretched back and opened my legs, ready for his hands to do their magic. His fingers played with my cunt. I was amazed that someone so young could possess such wonderful technique and dexterity with their hands. He started to go in and out of my pussy with relish. He put in two and then three fingers. *Ahhhh, yes, that feels good, don't stop. Continue.* My head fell back toward the floor. I felt as if I was doing "wheel," a yoga position where I stand on my hands and feet backward, and it felt divine. I let my cunt reach out to him to receive the pleasure he was giving me. My mind kept saying *Fuck me, fuck me,* until I started groaning out loud.

I looked down to see his wrist fucking my cunt with a ferocity that made me say, "Yes, do it, do it more, don't stop. Please fuck me more!" He obviously must have connected with my G-spot because all of a sudden a gush of fluid spurted up and out all over his hand, wrist, and arm. These type of orgasms are experienced more by mature women, who are more relaxed and in touch with themselves sexually. The

Mr. Handsome

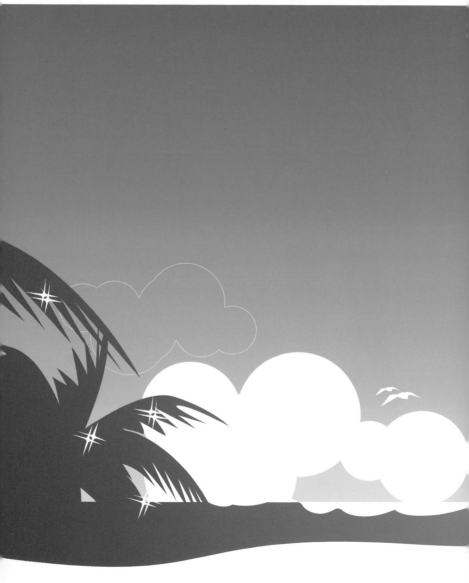

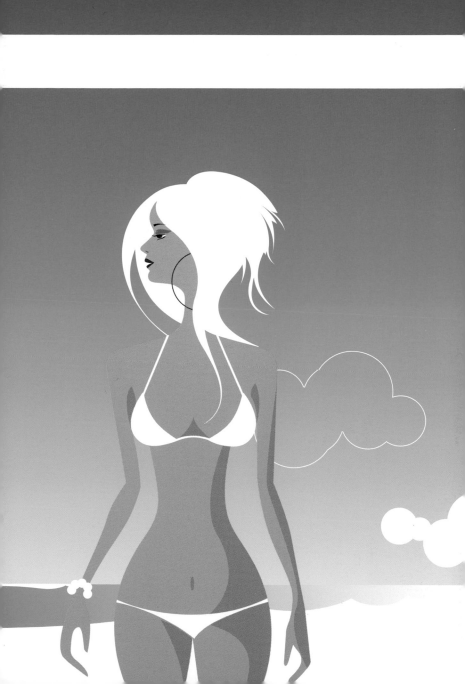

The girls and I were out one night having drinks. Adina, my best girlfriend, caught the eye of a tall, suave young man in his early thirties. He was wearing a beautiful Ermenegildo Zegna suit. Having known Adina for more than a decade, I knew that she had a soft spot for this type of look—sleek, sophisticated, and very James Bond.

Adina was a struggling author. She had one book in bookstores and had just signed a contract for her second. She wrote steamy sex stories and how-to books. She frequently temped as a receptionist to pay her rent. Adina was an exotic creature approaching fifty with long black hair, olive skin, and pensive dark eyes. She loved carrying giant pocketbooks and wearing skinny jeans with black suede boots. She could wear a garbage bag and look stunning. She ran through Central Park because it kept her gorgeous and was cheaper than a health club. You would never know by looking at her that she was one step away from the poorhouse. Adina had a penchant for power players. I didn't blame her. But eyeing someone in their thirties was a new experience for her.

I leaned over and whispered to Adina that a gorgeous young man was looking in her direction. Adina's feline head turned as her black hair trailed down her back with a curl. It was akin to watching a cat approach a saucer of milk. I thought, *Oh, God, girl, you are going to lap this right up.* As I watched Mr. Handsome, I thought he definitely was charming and pleasing to the eye. He was of Spanish descent with a bit of an accent. I have to say that accent made him drop-dead gorgeous. He had soft brown eyes and wore his hair casually parted in the middle and a little long behind his ears—he reminded me of Javier Bardem, who made me want to keel over, he was so hot. If she didn't want this guy, I would grab him in a heartbeat. He wore a crisp white shirt unbuttoned, exposing a bit of his sexy chest. He had a quiet way about him that was extremely appealing.

I noticed Mr. Handsome and Adina had their heads bent toward each other and were laughing. He bought her another Cosmopolitan. I thought, *That's it, we've lost her.* I must say they made a formidable couple. The two of them resembled exotic birds of paradise. At the end of the evening I asked Adina, "How'd ya do?"

"He gave me his number," she said with a smirk. Like this was a surprise to me.

A few days later Adina and I were going for a coffee in the Village.

"Do I look fat?" She asked me.

"No," I said.

"Does my hair need to be dyed?"

"Uh, no." I said, "Adina, what is up with you? You seem a bit edgy."

"I have a date with the South American hottie."

"Oh, Mr. Handsome? Pray tell, where are you going?" I asked. *This should be good,* I thought to myself.

He was taking her to an early dinner at Nobu, which was a restaurant in Manhattan featuring a whole new design in Japanese cuisine. Then they were going to the show called Absynthe. I had seen it; it resembled the Cirque du Soleil on crack. Very cool.

"So I don't get it, why so edgy?"

Adina was almost twenty years older than this young man. She was feeling a bit insecure about her age and how he might perceive her. Heaven forbid he saw a gray hair. Adina admitted to me that she felt a bit self-conscious going out with a younger man. Would he think she was too old? Would he notice the crow's-feet around her eyes? And what would he think of her body? It was in great shape, but she was fifty, not twenty. What if he thought she was too saggy? I reassured her that if he did, he was an asshole, but this didn't seem to be the case.

I tried to explain that the man was intrigued with her because of her maturity. She exuded style and sophistication. Many young cubs particularly like this. I told Adina that she had traveled all over the world and had one book out and another on the way. "Woman, you are a force to be reckoned with. You may find that both you and he have a lot in common." Sometimes cougars need to understand their own appeal to the younger man and have some faith in their own fabulousity. Adina could handle a power player, but one so young was new to her. I told her this was going to be the best thing for her and would fit into her independent lifestyle perfectly.

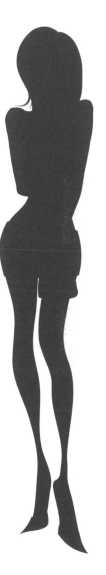

This seemed to work for Adina. She put on a stunning dress and pair of stilettos. A squirt of perfume and she was ready to go. Her hair was simply a lush mane of jaguar black. Her buzzer rang and Mr. Handsome asked for her to come downstairs. When she walked out the door, she was greeted by Mr. Handsome's car. Terrific. The driver opened the door and there he was with all his handsomeness waiting for her. She stepped in and sat down.

"Good evening." *Can I faint now?* she thought.

She slid into the car and showed her legs, tanned thanks to her tan-in-a-tube at home.

"Would you care for some wine?" he asked.

"That would be lovely," she replied.

Adina wondered if she could pour it all over herself and have him lick it off. Well, maybe later. He gave her a smile that could have melted the North Pole in a second. She was slightly stunned that someone of this age could be so appealing to her. It made her stomach feel funny. They sped down to Nobu. They were brought to a lovely table in the house and a single magnolia was perfectly placed in the middle of her plate. She had a feeling this wasn't by accident. He ordered a divine bottle of wine. He had so much style for a young man. Like so many cougars, she was surprised at how engaging he was to talk to.

Adina told me later that he was genuinely interested in her writing and wasn't put off by the fact that she was considered a sexpert. She could tell he was impressed by her accomplishments. He asked thoughtful questions, which was such a relief from some of the inane radio shows she had been featured on for her book tour. Adina found older men did not seem to give her the appreciation for her talent that this young man was displaying. She found it truly made her feel valued for who she was. I think this is the major appeal of young men for cougars. It is the driving factor for our current lifestyles.

"Give me details, Adina. What the hell is he like?" I asked. I was dying to know.

Adina was intrigued by how Mr. Handsome had landed here in the States. He had come here for school and ran his father's business, which had to do with imports and a bunch of other stuff. It turned out he kept a home in South America, another in South Beach, and a condo in Manhattan.

"Holy mackerel, Adina. How wonderful to be able to lead a life like that and at such a young age!" I exclaimed.

Adina was honest with him that talking money just wasn't her forte, but they seemed to do just fine. She actually felt she needed to talk about the age thing. It made her feel uncomfortable. She couldn't wrap her mind around the fact that he wanted to be with her. Didn't he want some twenty-year-old? He assured her that she had so much more to offer than a twenty-year-old and that was what he found alluring.

MR. HANDSOME—PART II

Adina sat at her computer trying to concentrate on the sex story she was writing. She had to admit she had been recently inspired by Mr. Handsome. She was so inspired she took time out to go lie on her bed and masturbate. People would laugh if they knew this was actually a writing technique that she used for ideas. Seriously, she didn't finish until she had at least four orgasms. Adina found each orgasm brought a new idea. Hey, it worked for her. She was on idea number four when her cell phone tinkled.

"Hello." It was Mr. Handsome. There was no mistaking that silken voice. God, it went straight to her cunt. "How are you?" he asked.

"I'm fine. Thanks for a lovely evening last week."

"I was wondering if you would like to have a picnic on the beach?"

"Uh, that would be nice, but isn't it a little cold for that right now?"

"I'll figure something out. Shall I pick you up tomorrow around ten in the morning?"

She couldn't imagine what he was thinking, but agreed to meet him anyway.

Saturday morning I called Adina. "What are you doing?" I asked.

"Running around trying to figure how to dress for a picnic on the beach in New York in February."

"Oh, that's all? Adina, you have to admit you would never have some old geezer ask you to do something like this. Why don't you wear your standard uniform—jeans, boots, and black parka?" Done, no big deal. I rolled my eyes in disbelief at the thought of an accomplished woman getting in a tizzy over a date with a thirty-two-year-old. Give me a break.

Her buzzer rang at exactly 10 A.M. The driver opened the door and there was Mr. Handsome in a pair of jeans and a leather jacket. I told Adina that this man made David Beckham look like chopped liver. As she slid onto the seat, he put his hand around the back of her neck and pulled her over to give her a deep tongue kiss. Jeez.

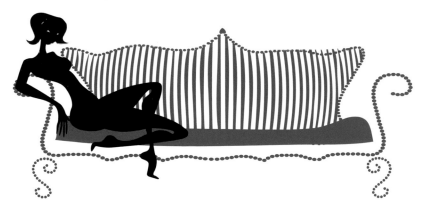

One enticing kiss after another, he worked his way down between her breasts and softly kissed along her stomach.

Oh, my God. This is heaven, she thought. He was so fucking gorgeous—so tantalizing.

He made his way to the top of her jeans. He popped open the snap and looked up at her with a mischievous look in his eyes. Then he undid her zipper. Her hips naturally tilted up toward his face. He continued to work his way down her groin, inhaling her smell as he did. He pulled them down with a quick jerk. Adina loved it. *Yeah, this works,* she thought. He pulled off her boots. *Fuck the stewardess, fuck any turbulence, let's create a little of our own.* She grabbed him and flipped herself on top. She grabbed his neck and kissed him with all her might. She was in control now. She matched his kisses with her own, holding him, grabbing his head to steady both of them for the deepness of it.

Later, I asked Adina to give me all the details on the plane. She told me the plane started to rumble for takeoff. A smooth voice over the intercom stated, "Please fasten your seat belts." Mr. Handsome grabbed a belt from behind them and wrapped it around the two of them and clicked them in. Adina was laughing and kissing him at the same time. As the plane roared into the air, Adina and Mr. Handsome roared into each other. To be so physically united with someone cosmically while thundering into space was a mind-blowing experience. She had never quite been kissed in such a manner. Let's say she liked it.

Once the plane leveled off they lay back in each other's arms to catch their breath. Adina said, "Well, this beats picking up my laundry this morning." Mr. Handsome laughed as he poured them some wine. Mr. Handsome looked at her and stated, "Speaking of that, you may need a few things for where we are going. Let's take care of it when we land, shall we?"

Adina smiled weakly and wondered what planet she had landed on.

MR. HANDSOME AND ADINA GO SHOPPING

"So what did you do once you got there? What was it like? And for God's sake, what was he like?" I asked.

Three and a half hours later Adina was blinded by the sun streaming through the plane windows. Adina looked at Mr. Handsome and asked, "Okay, where are we?"

"Florida. South Beach, to be exact," he replied.

Of course we are, she thought, *and here I am wearing winter boots and a parka. Great.*

They stepped off the plane as the hot sun assaulted them. Adina felt beads of sweat pop out between her breasts. A champagne-colored limousine awaited them. Mr. Handsome opened the door for her and led her in. The coolness of the car calmed her skin, but not her mind. Mr. Handsome took off his jacket and instructed the driver to take them to a department store. Adina's eyes bugged slightly out of her head.

"What size dress and shoe are you?" he asked Adina.

Mr. Handsome got on his cell phone and dialed the store. "Hello, Diane. I am here with a friend. She is a size-eight dress and shoe. She will need everything for a fabulous weekend here. We will see you in a few minutes.

"Do you do this all the time?" She asked, wondering how many women he had done this with.

"Actually, no, Diane is my own personal shopper, but she can do anything." He smiled.

They arrived at the department store, where Mr. Handsome held her hand and led her upstairs to a suite of beautifully designed rooms. A tall, perfectly coiffed blond woman dressed in Chanel greeted them. Clearly, this was Diane. As I listened to Adina tell me about this, all I could think of was, this was the kind of behavior you would expect from a seasoned CEO in his late fifties—she had landed a spectacular young man. I was a tad envious.

Mr. Handsome sat back with a smile on his face. It was rare to be with a woman who knew herself so well. Her ability to take command of a situation was admirable and quite sexy. This is one of the main attractions of dating a cougar.

Diane had taken the liberty of having a light lunch prepared for them and had it wheeled in. They dined on a salad with small finger sandwiches. By the time they were done, Diane brought in a rack of stunning pieces of clothing. Adina clapped her hands in delight.

"Would you like me to stay and assist you?" Diane asked.

"I think we will be just fine," Mr. Handsome replied. "I'll call you if we need anything."

Adina raised her eyebrows and thought, *okey-dokey.* She had never been with a man who had such a smooth confidence and ability to take command of a situation for her. Most of the time people just expected her to be the one in control. This man knew when to step in with style and panache and he was in his early thirties. She found these same components hot and sexy in a man. She found it went straight to her clit.

She flipped open a box of bright yellow stiletto sandals. She inhaled the smell of leather deeply as she slipped them over her chili-pepper-manicured toes. She grabbed a sheer little yellow number and ran into the dressing room to slip it on. She took off her underwear, since they were a mess anyway, and threw them in the trash. She fluffed her hair and walked out to show Mr. Handsome. Adina later told me she had gone back to being petrified about how this young stud would view her body. Would he be disappointed when he saw her naked?

When she looked into his eyes she was struck by the intense way he looked at her. He looked at her as if he was going to devour her and worship everything about her. It was as if it was her and only her that mattered to him. Wow, what a heady feeling.

"Come here," he said to her.

Slowly she walked over to him as the silkiness of the fabric brushed against her thighs. Their eyes never left each other. She walked directly to him and stood about an inch away. He reached forward and slipped his hand behind her leg above her knee.

"I like this," he said looking directly into her eyes. She felt something hit her deep within. He slid his hand further up the backside of her leg. She moved in closer so his knee was between hers. His hand moved to the soft inside of her thigh. Her mouth opened slightly as she wet her lower lip with her tongue.

"Tell me if you want me to stop," he said.

"I don't want you to stop," she whispered.

Feeling the velvetiness of her thigh, he continued to run his hand up her leg. Their eyes continued to penetrate each other. He felt her ass and then slowly ran his fingers from the back to the front of her cunt. He pulled his hand out and looked at the wetness all over it. He brought it to his face and smelled it. He looked back up at her and licked his hand. He took his middle finger and sucked it with his mouth. He then returned his finger to her cunt and submerged it between her thighs, plunging into her. She put her hand against the wall to brace herself. He then put two fingers inside her. Slowly he brought them in and out of her pussy lips. He then put them in deep and rotated them back and forth. Adina held on as a breath escaped her. She closed her eyes for a moment to take in the intensity she was experiencing. She looked back at him as he took his fingers and went in for the kill. Rapidly, he shoved his fingers up and down inside her. She held on for dear life as she felt the heat start to build. Her head bent down as the electrical charges shot through her clit. *It is coming, it is coming, oh Jesus, it is here!* Great jolts of current shot through her pussy, through her cunt, down her legs, and up her ass. She gritted her teeth trying not to scream her brains out. She came and gushed all over his hand and down his arm. She squeezed her legs as the spasms ceased. Her panting slowed down as she continued to steady herself against the wall. Her breathing was still heavy as she looked at him and smiled. He grabbed her and pulled her to his lap. He kissed her passionately as she wrapped her arms around his neck. They stayed like that for a few minutes and prepared themselves for the rest of the day.

MR. HANDSOME
ON THE BEACH

"Okay, so then what happened?" I asked.

"Well, his house is in South Beach Home. I've been with players before, but not this age and I have to tell you it changed the dynamic and threw me off my game a bit," she told me.

Mr. Handsome brought her inside. Adina felt as if she were walking through a spread in *Architectural Digest*. Everything was clean, fresh, white, and expansive. She just loved it. He brought her to the master bedroom, which was to die for. There was a little dressing room where she could hang her new clothes. It had a makeup table and lights so she could sit and beautify, not to mention her own private bathroom.

"Why don't you put on your bathing suit and we will go to the beach?" he said.

"That sounds great." Adina replied.

She rummaged through the bags and found a Calvin Klein slate-gray two-piece bathing suit. She couldn't wait to put it on. She looked at herself in the mirror and was pleased that she could still wear a two-piece bathing suit and pull it off wonderfully. Thank

God her stomach was looking flat. She hated having these doubts and insecurities. She put on some black flip-flops, a big straw hat, and a paisley chiffon cover-up. Yipee! She walked out into the bedroom and almost had a heart attack. There was Mr. Handsome in all his handsomeness wearing nothing but a small pair of black trunks and a pair of leather sandals. His tanned skin was smooth and contained perfectly shaped pecs, a six-pack for abs, and strong long legs. His package wasn't looking too bad, either.

"Holy fuck, Adina. Do you have any pictures of this? What was the cock like? Tell me about the cock," I asked.

"Are you ready?" he asked quietly.

Was she ready? She was ready to fuck the shit out of him, but thought she should try to have some sort of control and not give the impression of being a total nymphomaniac.

"I'm very ready."

He took her hand and led her down the winding staircase. They walked out the French doors into a living paradise.

"Oh my God," Adina exclaimed.

There was a stunning pool with a bubbling waterfall, sumptuous pillows were resting on outrageous chaise lounges, and a Jacuzzi was waiting on the side. Palm trees, shrubs, and bird-of-paradise flowers were everywhere. And then there was the beach, a private beach with sand so white it blinded her. Mr. Handsome led her down the stairs to the beach. He put his arm around her waist and kissed her.

"I'm so glad you are here. Let's take a walk on the beach, shall we?" he asked.

Could he make her feel any more wanted or appreciated? Adina had gone through a lot of men in her lifetime and recently she had gone through a drought. She knew someone fantastic when she met him. Mr. Handsome was truly divine. They took a luxurious stroll down the beach with the sun on their backs, hand in hand, with the water splashing over their feet. When they returned they lay by the pool while a butler brought them some seltzer water. Mr. Handsome told her about his family and what it was like leading a life of luxury in South America and the expectations his father had for him to run the family's business. She told him about her life as a writer and the challenges of writing about sex all the time. They talked about anything and everything—food, movies, fashion, and even fingernail polish. He liked red, by the way.

"Feeling hungry?" he asked.

"Famished."

"Let's get ready for dinner, shall we?"

"Absolutely."

The bathroom in her dressing room was magnificent. Adina stood with showers spraying her from every angle. All the salt was washed from every crevice in her body. There was a splendid array of soaps and potions for her to play with. After she showered she put a golden lotion all over her body that left a bit of a sheen to her skin. She sprayed herself with perfume, slipped on her new shoes and dress. She walked out to Mr. Handsome, who was wearing his standard fitted white shirt and black pants, no socks, and slip-on black shoes. James Bond, eat your heart out. The driver opened the door to whisk them away to dinner. They arrived at The Tides Hotel. It is a grand 1936 art deco hotel that has been restored to its original beauty.

Mr. Handsome guided her to the elevators,

which were parfaits of crystal elegance. Once the doors closed he placed her in the corner and kissed her deeply. She found his cock with her hand and squeezed it tight. She was happy to see the man was just to her satisfaction. The elevator doors opened and he led her down the hallway. When they reached the end, he took out the key and opened a door to a suite. The room was a private oasis in shades of warm sandy tones. The entire wall of the room was taken up by a window overlooking the beach and the ocean. It even had a telescope for star watching. But there were candles everywhere and gardenias as well. The air was fragrant with the scent of flowers, candles, and the sea. The windows were floor length and had been opened with a table situated so they could overlook the ocean.

"I thought you might enjoy a private dinner," he said to her.

"Yes, it is a bit different from a noisy bistro in New York, isn't it?" *What a treat*, she thought.

A waiter quietly knocked on the door and wheeled in a cart of sumptuous goodies all hidden underneath silver domes. Mr. Handsome held out a chair for Adina. The waiter put a napkin on her lap and pulled out a fabulous bottle of champagne. Adina took a moment to take it all in: this handsome

man, the ocean air brushing against her face, and
even the plush chair she was sitting on. She didn't
take things for granted. She had come from humble
beginnings in New Hampshire as a kid, so she was
grateful when things were good. *This is better than
good, this is fantabulous.*

She looked up and saw Mr. Handsome smiling
at her while holding her hand. He picked up the
champagne flute with his other hand.

"To the most stunning woman I have ever met,"
he said to her.

She felt the heat rise to her face as she picked up
her own glass. "Thank you for a stupendous day." He
was so handsome, so vibrant, and so full of life. They
then ate a tasty meal of sautéed lobster, scallops, and
shrimps.

When they finished Mr. Handsome pulled out a
little dome and took the top off. Underneath was a
shell made of hard chocolate stuffed with a chocolate
mousse.

When she told me later, I said to Adina that I
would have smeared that dessert all over him.

Mr. Handsome slowly picked up a silver
dessertspoon and looked at her with those warm
brown eyes of his. His lips slowly smiled as he dipped
the tip of the spoon in the whipped confection. He

brought the spoon up to her lips for her to eat. She did so slowly. He did this again. Then Adina took her finger and dipped it into the little chocolate shell and scooped out a dollop of chocolate mousse. She then got up from the table, sat in Mr. Handsome's lap, and smeared it over his lips. She then took her time licking his top lip and then sucked in his lower lip as if she was going to eat it. His tongue came darting out and into the depths of her mouth. *Is it possible to fall in love with a person's tongue?* Never had Adina experienced a tongue that could actually rule her body by its erotic tenacity. She took it in with anticipation.

She stood up so she could straddle him. She had always wanted to do this to someone at the dinner table. She wrapped her arms around him and went in for a luscious kiss. She knew how to use her mouth, too. She put her hand down and unbuckled his belt. His hands were on either side of her face, holding her as he kissed her right back. She pulled out his cock and stood up a little. She was only wearing a little G-string, so she pulled it aside as she lowered herself on his rock-solid cock. It was difficult on the legs to maintain this position, but Adina found that it positioned her pussy right over the cock, so she could have a deep insertion. In other words, it made for a

was a believer in cougar power.

Adina and I were walking down the street the following week.

"See, I told you he was going to be fun. *And* he has a cock—a great cock!" I grinned.

"I am just stunned by the whole thing. The funny thing is, I want more."

"Darling, there is nothing better than a hot young man to get the juices flowing," I mused.

"Uh-huh, yeah, uh-huh," Adina said.

TYPES OF COUGARS

→**Power Cougar**—Think of Condoleezza Rice. This woman is a power player in the boardroom. She wears her own power suit, is highly educated, and holds her own with the big boys. She may be well known in Wall Street, Madison Avenue, or Washington, D.C. But you will not see her with her boy toy in public. She is discreet about her dalliances due to her high position.

→**Intellectual Cougar**—This woman is highly educated and accomplished. Think of Gloria Steinem or Arianna Huffington. She is frequently on the talk show circuit discussing her latest philosophy or book.

→**The Unexpected Cougar**—This is the last person you would expect to have an affair with a younger man. She is quiet and demure, maybe a librarian or administrative assistant. She may find that young man from South America and love to engage in hot pursuit behind closed doors outside of work.

→**The Divorcée Cougar**—This woman has just been through a rough divorce after a devoted marriage of double-digit years. She just wants to have fun with no attachments whatsoever.

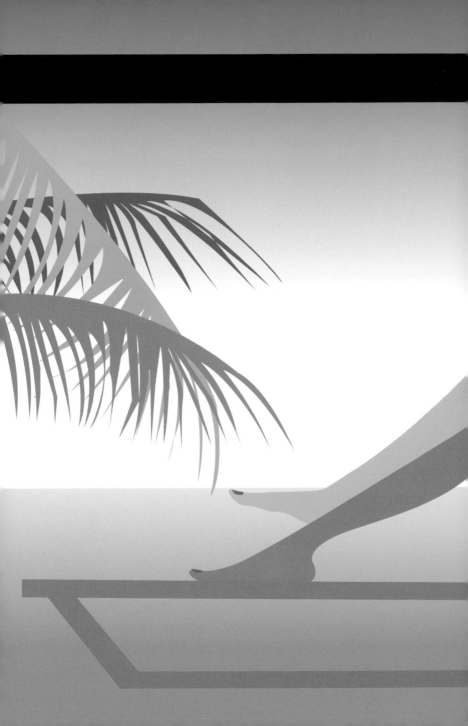

Piña Colada Man

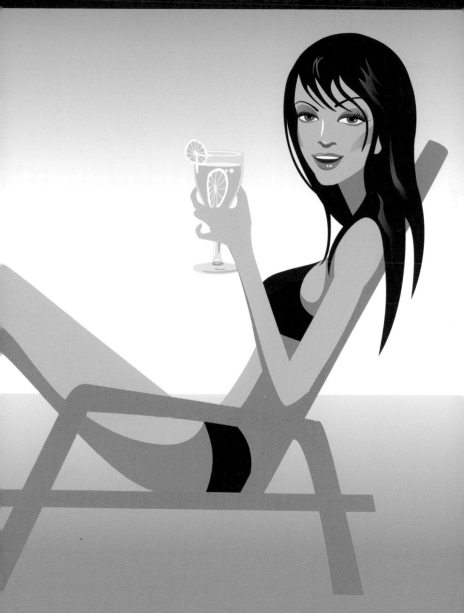

Sam had to be the most divine cougar because she was so on top of her game. She was forty-nine, part Hungarian and part French. She had luminous skin with dark green pensive eyes. She was 5'9" with long, long legs, and always donned three-inch heels. She wore her auburn hair shoulder length with golden highlights. She had been married once, to her best friend, but it only lasted a year. She found she preferred him as her buddy. Sam was a television producer in Manhattan for a hot sitcom. She worked hard and she played hard. She enjoyed being single at this stage in her life. She didn't want anyone tying her down. She once told me that she enjoyed going home at night and having her place all to herself. Sam called me and said she was planning a Caribbean cruise to tan that lovely body of hers. The cruise was meant for singles. All I could think was *God help those men on that boat.* This woman didn't mess around.

I sat on the edge of her bed as Sam packed her Louis Vuitton luggage with some of the most gorgeous bikinis you could imagine. She was waxed, buffed, and trimmed prior to the trip.

"So did you get a Brazilian?" I asked her.

"Of course, darling."

"Do they really wax your asshole?"

"Yes, they do. I mean, you never know who is going to be back there."

I thought the woman had a point. Waxing was all the rage these days and men seemed to love it, particularly the younger ones. I decided to make a note to look into getting one for myself the next time I had a date with a hottie.

She booked one of the finer rooms with a gorgeous view of the ocean with her own private deck. Go, girl, go. The afternoon Sam arrived she promptly went to her room, got settled, and then threw off her clothes to put on a little yellow bikini covered by a stunning chiffon number that just grazed her buttocks. She brushed her hair, slipped on her gold metallic shoes, and put on a large pair of black sunglasses. She strode onto the deck of the ship as if she were walking in a runway show at the height of Fashion Week.

Sam selected a blue canvas lounge chair by the pool overlooking the ocean. *This will certainly do.* She lay back, took off her chiffon sheath, and kicked off her gold sandals. She sighed deeply and closed her

eyes. *Yes, this is perfect.* Now for a little refreshment.
A waiter came by and took her order. "I'll have a piña
colada," she stated. She got comfortable and sipped
her drink while soaking in the hot sun. She closed her
eyes and dozed off.

Sam was nicely groggy when she opened her eyes
to the sight of a Greek god rising from the pool's
depths. He must have been well over six feet, his skin
was bronzed, and his body, oh God, that body. Every
slope of every muscle was flawless in its shape. His
pecs were in exact proportion from working out,
not too much and not too little. His aureolae were
chocolate brown from the sun. Sam's eyes grazed
along his chest, and down his stomach. He wore black
stretch swim trunks that just skimmed his gorgeous
hips. She wanted to run her tongue right above the
band just covering his hips. The water trickled down,
teasing her mind. And then the package, can we talk
about the package?

Oh, fuck, I am truly going to wet myself, Sam
thought.

His cock formed a faultless bulge in that sweet
little bathing suit. Sam dropped her sunglasses down
her nose and let her eyes make contact with his as he
stepped out of the pool to pick up a towel. He had a
slow smile as he looked at her.

She smiled back. "Care to join me?"

"Sure, what are you drinking?"

"Piña colada."

"We'll have two piña coladas," he told the waiter. He brushed back his wet hair. Sam thought about running her hands through it and grabbing it hard. Her mind was working overtime and her bathing suit was getting moist without her even having been in the pool.

They lay back in the warm afternoon sun and had a lovely time just chatting amiably. He was a trader on Wall Street, in his early thirties, and used to a very social career wining and dining his clients. He was frustrated with some of the young girls he had dated. They all wanted to get married and seemed to look at him as a meal ticket. As he talked to Sam, he stated it was refreshing to meet a sophisticated woman like herself who knew who she was and had lived so many interesting experiences. Sam stretched her legs like a cat. She felt appreciated and knew that this young man would be able to offer her openness, intelligence, and a high-testosterone body. This suited her needs nicely at this stage in the game. She found a young man refreshing. No archaic bullshit such as what she might encounter with someone in his sixties who had to have his dinner at 6:30 P.M. every night.

After another piña colada, he suggested she roll over and he would put some suntan lotion on her back. "Oh yes, certainly, that would be good." She made herself comfortable as she felt him untie her bikini top. *This boy doesn't waste any time,* she grinned to herself. She felt lotion pour slowly down her back and arched just a tad to meet it. He had large, warm hands that moved with strength against her skin. He took his time kneading her muscles to the consistency of butter. He massaged every notch of her spine. He pressed her shoulders and moved down her arms and then her sides. He moved down her buttocks and worked the mounds of her ass.

She thought, *Jesus, between him and the sun I don't care what he does to me at this point.*

She felt him go down the crack of her ass. She couldn't help but think of Steven Tyler in Aerosmith singing, *Love on an elevator, living it up and I'm going down.* Just as he hit the ground floor she felt his finger slip under her bathing suit and into her pussy. He worked his way in, twisting his finger in and out so discreetly that no one knew what he was doing. If they did, Sam could have given a hoot by that time.

Just as she was about to give herself to the Sun God of the Caribbean, she felt his warm lips on her ear.

"Follow me," he said.

She opened her eyes and looked up. He took her hand and led her to a cabana behind the pool. They stepped into the shaded tent, which featured a little sofa with pillows spread all over it. She sat on it and in one fell swoop slid his marvelous bathing suit to the floor. As she did this his cock slipped into her mouth. Her coral nails glittered around him and her other hand pulled his scrotum down. Sam had learned a few things from hanging with young men. She dragged one fingernail underneath his cock toward the tip. She had learned that this drives a man crazy. She did this while continuing to pull his scrotum down in her other hand. She eased her tongue in between the little crevice and followed it with a suck of the tip. She went to the base and tea-bagged his balls (sucking both at one time). She lapped underneath his cock all the way up again. *Lap, lap, lap.* She lubed it up with her spit and twisted her hand up and down slowly as she began to deep-throat his cock. She continued to suck, pull, and twist to her heart's delight. His strong legs supported him as his head tilted back in pleasure. This man infused her with inspiration. She wanted as much of him as she possibly could get.

He pushed her back against the sofa. Their skin was slick with lotion and they slid into place. The sofa was cool against her back as she opened her legs naturally to welcome him in. His cock was a hefty size and caused her to gasp as he filled her. It was just the right size for her and she pushed her hips against it to show she was going to fuck him as much as he was going to fuck her. It seemed they were in definite agreement about this subject.

Once they had had their way with each other, Sam made him sit on the edge of the sofa and straddled him with her feet on the floor. She placed her hands on his shoulders and looked directly into his eyes. She liked having her feet on the floor because this way she could command how she rode him. She was used to taking control sexually and had no inhibitions about it. She didn't want a man who did, either. Young men seemed to be up to the task and physically their stamina could match Sam's. This is no easy feat, but it is a classic scenario with a young man–older woman pair.

She started slow by going up and down, feeling the fullness of his girth. She sat on him firmly and rode her hips into his. Then she quickened the pace so that she could rub her clit against his hardness and make herself come. She waited for the tingling heat to start. When she felt the first spasms start to erupt, she dug her nails into his flesh and bit her teeth down so she wouldn't make any noise in the canvas cabana. She rocked, she rubbed, deeper, harder and there it was. The heat radiated up and out of her. *Eureka!*

Afterward, Sam thought, *God, I love piña coladas.*

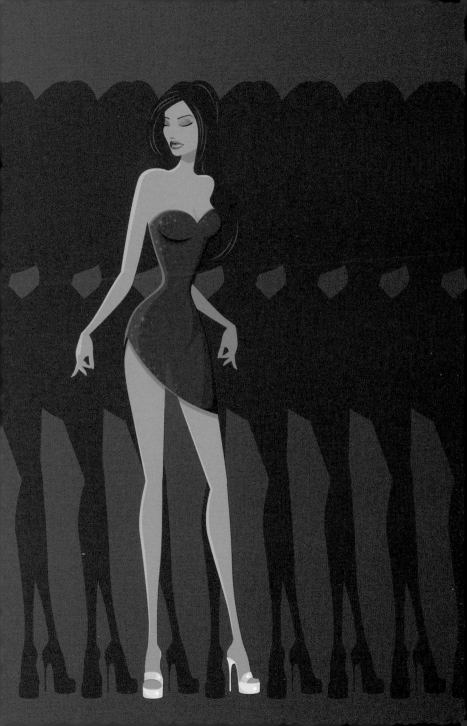

The Bodacious Lula

I worked for a time with Lula, who was a bodacious Puerto Rican babe in her thirties. She must have weighed about 250 pounds and had breasts the size of two giant melons. But she loved her sexiness and dressed with total sensuality. It made me happy to see this. I knew she'd probably like to enjoy herself when she got naked with someone. One day she came in wearing a hot pink form-fitting top that showed her ample bosom. Each day she wore a different-colored thong. When she bent over, the crack of her ass greeted you with a good-sized tattoo. Lula was known as a BBW (big beautiful woman). There was no missing Lula.

Lula called me over to her desk one day to look at her computer. She had pulled up a page on MySpace that showed this hot, young Caribbean man. She had a profile on MySpace, with friends and all sorts of information about herself on it. She literally had a portfolio of pictures hot young men had sent to her. This is a whole new world that I'm not really involved in—it seems to be more of a venue for younger people. I know it was a turnoff when I looked at one young man's profile and it featured tons of pictures of him drinking with his friends and girls making out with each other. This is not the sort of thing a cougar wants to see, but she sure does want to see hot pictures of hot men. I told Lula to show me more. Hey, they were her friends, not mine.

Lula's Caribbean studmuffin was 6'3" and had a massive chest. He wore his tattoos proudly. Lula was a great example of the younger cougar. She wanted a serious relationship, but didn't mind riding a hot young stud while she was searching. Photo after photo featured a hot young stallion whose testosterone was fully stocked. One of the best shots was a side view of his tongue. My eyebrows lifted as I looked at its length. He was a whopping eighteen years of age and looked like an absolute powerhouse.

Lula had to take a call one day that was obviously important to her. I listened as she flirted shamelessly. Her accent clipped her words as if she was giving him quick flicks of her tongue. I figured she must be talking to Powerhouse. I watched as she brushed her hair over her shoulder while talking on her cell. The girl was definitely inflamed. *Oh boy.* I just rolled my eyes.

Lula informed me that she was meeting Powerhouse after Valentine's Day when he got off work. He was a private weight trainer. Thus the arm muscles that went on forever. I wondered what his other muscles might look like. Lula was so excited she looked as if she might cream in her panties before she even met him. Frankly, I didn't blame the woman.

Lula dated her young stud for a couple of months. Every time she saw him she came in the day after looking like a soft marshmallow floating on air. I asked her what it was that was so hot about Powerhouse. She said he would just look at her and it would drive her crazy. He would stare and caress every inch of her body with his eyes. She said it made her feel like a million bucks, not to mention a total sensuous woman.

Lula usually had Powerhouse come to her place. I find this is more common for cougars. Cougars are older and have a desire to have a nice home. Their home is their haven where they regenerate and spend time reading, painting, working, lounging, cooking, or taking a nice bubble bath. Younger men frequently don't have a sense of style in home decorating. In fact, they may live with roommates and the place is a sty. This is hardly romantic for a cougar. She may suggest he come over for dinner and then have him for dessert. Whipped cream anyone?

One evening Lula told me that she was taking a shower after they had just had sex. In the middle of her shower, Powerhouse ripped back the shower curtain and just stared at her. He stood there without a stitch of clothing on him and his cock reaching out and calling out to her. She couldn't have felt more wanted. He pulled her out of the shower and threw her on the bed. No towel, nothing. Water flew all over the place. He started to put that beautiful tongue to work. Lula said he put it everywhere. She lolled on the bed as that burning penis worked its way over her breasts. He smothered his face between her tits. She laughed as she smooshed them to envelop his head. He wiggled down and ran his tongue over the rolls of her side, working his way around to her ass and flipping her on her belly in the process. This tongue-lashing was equivalent to a hot oil massage. A low growl worked its way out of her throat.

He took his time. She loved how he paid special attention to kissing and sucking her pussy lips. He would smack her with a loud kiss down there in between licks. Powerhouse would flatten his tongue and give big long licks from one end of her pussy to her clit. She loved that. Gradually he worked his way to her ass. He had a lot to work with and wanted to savor every succulent suckle. He took little bites of her sweet spot, the perfect place where you want to spank someone. Lula, by this time, had gone into a hypnotic trance. Just as she thought it couldn't get any better Powerhouse tickled her butthole with his tongue. He spread her cheeks and licked her rim. She gave herself with total abandon. She had found over the years that she had grown to really enjoy anal sex and open herself up to it. This stud was a force to be reckoned with. What was even better was he didn't stop. He went in and out, teasing her hole to open for him. He slipped his finger in her pussy, first one, then two. Once he was in he started to swirl the two fingers around back and forth, first clockwise and then counterclockwise. Lula's growl became fiercer.

Powerhouse reached up inside her walls and found her G-spot. He tickled her spongy spot while continuing her anal tongue-lashing. If a woman feels comfortable with her partner she can really let loose in this position. Finally it was as if Mount Vesuvius was erupting. She gushed a clear fluid all over his face, leaving the smell of sweet clover. This kind of orgasm will not stain the sheets, my friends. It is also one of the most intense orgasms a woman can have.

I laughed when Lula told me about her orgasm. The first time it happened to me I knew what it was, but it was still a surprise. I was a little embarrassed in that it just went all over my partner's hand, arm, and the bed. Then I said, "Oh, who gives a fuck? It means I was having a damn good one, so why should I be embarrassed?" Then I became proud that I could squirt as well as a man, if not better. How cool was that?

Lula told me that Powerhouse wasted no time at all. He got up on his knees and pulled her to his cock. He plunged in at the perfect moment. Lula was now growling at full force. He did something that felt as if he was churning his cock around inside her. Powerhouse was into pounding. It felt as if he was going to go right through to her brain. She felt somewhat dazed. He gave her ass a slap in between for good measure. She was surprised that one little slap could go straight to her clit. Whoa. When he came, Lula was not on this planet anymore. She was in outer space, floating on an orgasmic tapestry carpet.

Lula lay there semiconscious. Powerhouse had a training session to go to, so he slipped on his sneakers, workout pants, and a T-shirt. He gave her

a peck on the cheek and said, "So long, babe."
Lula rolled over and pulled her comforter
up around her neck. She snuggled in
while Ginger, her dog, jumped up
and found her place by Lula's feet.
She circled around with a snort.
Lula had the best snooze of her life,
and so did Ginger, by the way.

BEST PLACES FOR COUGARS TO HUNT FOR CUBS

→ Health club
→ Yoga class
→ Grocery store
→ Home Depot
→ Sports bars
→ Bars that feature rock bands
→ Any bar
→ Puma sports store
→ Sneaker shops
→ Sports events
→ Restaurants
→ Hair salon
→ Tanning salon

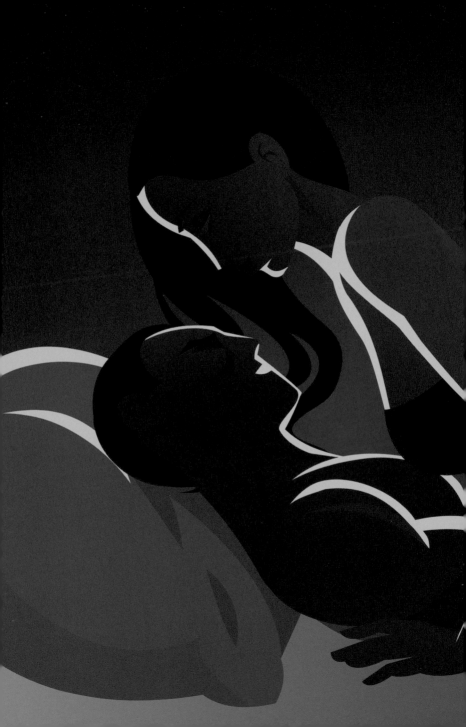

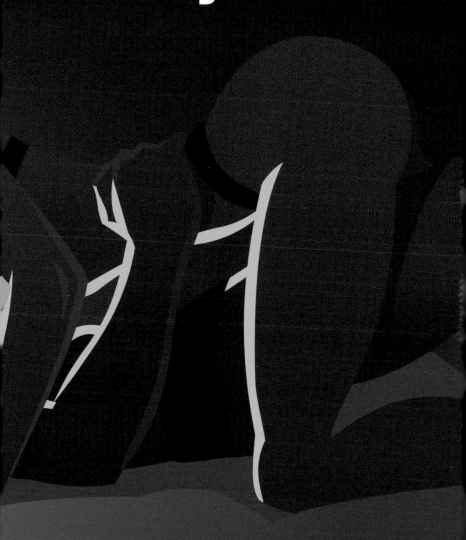

Billy Dee

Marlene was a friend of mine who was a therapist and had just turned forty. She worked at a methadone clinic in Boston. I couldn't fathom this stunning woman working in such a tough environment. It kind of made my skin crawl. She always seemed so cool and collected. She wore her auburn hair shoulder length and possessed luminosity about her that I assumed was from her spiritual life. There was something about her that made her seem as if she was always walking an inch above the ground. I found her simply fascinating.

Marlene and I were having lunch one day, discussing the men in our lives. We had both gone through divorces. Marlene shared with me that she met someone at work in the clinic. This was rare because you don't come across too many male social workers; they're mostly women. But this guy was about thirty and looked like the actor Billy Dee Williams in his younger days. *Not bad,* I thought. Marlene flicked her hair over her shoulder and said he was a really cool guy.

She'd been in the cafeteria one day, contemplating whether to have the pasta or a tuna sandwich. She heard this honey-infused voice say, "The pasta looks great." When she looked to her side she was a bit taken aback. Here was a fine-looking, tall, mocha-skinned man just looking at her. She shook her head and brilliantly replied, "What?"

"The pasta looks good," he stated with a friendly smile.

"Oh yeah, umm, but it's carbs," she said dumbly.

"Well, you don't look like you have to worry about it," he replied.

"Thanks. Do you work here?" she queried in disbelief.

"Yes, I am working at the men's treatment center. You?" he asked.

"I work at the methadone clinic."

"You know, I have so many questions about that. May I join you for lunch?" he asked.

Marlene continued to be stunned. Who meets a gorgeous man at the methadone clinic cafeteria? It was a freak of nature in her book. They found they had a lot to talk about and started to meet for lunch on a regular basis.

Marlene found him so easy to talk to. Billy Dee, as she called him, was from the South and had this special politeness to him. She hadn't had the pleasure of a man's company in such a long time, so this was quite the treat. One day he asked if she would like to go the movies. Again, she was surprised, not expecting it. She wasn't sure if this was an official date. She wasn't even sure she remembered *how* to date, since she had become so accustomed to being alone and single.

Marlene went a little crazy getting ready. Then she tried to calm herself by saying this wasn't a date. When they met in the parking lot, Marlene was struck by Billy Dee's smooth swagger. He wore a simple polo shirt and freshly pressed chinos, but he looked so handsome. He really did look like a movie star. As they sat through the movie, she couldn't help but notice the heat from his shoulder emanating through to hers. They went out for dinner afterward and Marlene found it was so easy to be with this man. They walked through the neighborhood, which featured spectacular oak trees lining the streets. As they looked up at the moon through the branches, he kissed her softly on the lips. It was sweet and lingering. Marlene thought she might melt right there in the middle of the sidewalk.

Marlene hadn't been courted in a long time. She couldn't help but wonder how she, a white divorcée entering her forties, was dating a younger African-American clinician. She chose to think: *Whatever.* It was a bit overwhelming, but she was at a stage in her life where she could appreciate what was being presented to her and let it unfold naturally. After several more lunches and movies, Billy Dee invited

Marlene to his apartment for dinner. She hadn't had a man cook her dinner in forever. This sort of thing was so old it was new for her. God, what would she wear, what should she bring him? Flowers? Wine? Dessert? Should she shave her legs? Put on her French perfume from Barney's? Wear a thong? A dress? Jeans?

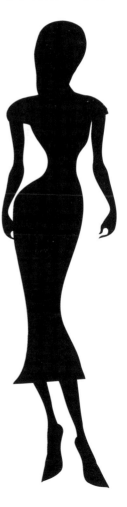

Marlene was one of these gorgeous, intelligent women who have a terrible time meeting men. This seems to be a common dilemma for mature, sophisticated women. There are a lot of hound dogs out there and she had had bad experiences with men drinking too much on a first date, lying about being single, and just wanting sex. It was very disappointing for her. She lived her life to the fullest, but sometimes this was a real drag. This whole experience with Billy Dee was totally unexpected. She never thought she would meet someone at work, someone who was so different from anyone she

It was an elegant room in warm, earthy tones with a soft light on the bureau. He lit a simple candle. Marlene's experience with men had proven that they either didn't have any furniture or lived like animals. This was not the case here, and she felt relieved. Billy Dee gently guided her to the bed. He took the time to look at her and held her face in his hands. He kissed each eyelid, her forehead, and then her nose. He made every moment so special. It was as if God had plucked this man down from heaven just for her. He kissed her mouth, found her tongue, and invited it to join his. She unbuttoned his shirt. His chest was velvety to her touch. She kissed the side of his neck. His lips found her bare shoulders. He untied her dress where it was knotted behind her neck. The two front panels fell to her waist. He ran his hands down her shoulders and around the sides of her breasts, cupping them and then kissing them. He looked into her eyes as he ran his fingers over her nipples, back and forth, back and forth. They stood to attention and alerted her juices to flow freely.

Marlene followed suit by sliding his shirt off his shoulders and onto the floor. She unbuckled his belt and unzipped his pants. She ran her hand over the front of him and felt a formidable cock waiting for her underneath. *Oh, goody,* she thought. He returned

FAMOUS COUGARS

→Tina Turner
→Cher
→Madonna
→Demi Moore
→Geena Davis
→Halle Berry
→Mae West
→Ivana Trump
→Susan Sarandon
→Kim Cattrall
→Cameron Diaz
→Carol Burnett

the favor by pulling off her dress and thong. He laughed as he purposely threw it on the floor with his shirt. They both laughed. She was now naked and wanted him to join her, so she slid his pants over his hips and let them add to the pile of clothes gathering on the floor. She was pleased that he was sans underwear. This was getting better by the minute.

They were both naked and rolled into each other's arms. They inhaled each other and kissed deeply. There is something to be said about taking one's time to get to know one another. Not all cougars are nymphomaniacs, jumping into sex every two minutes. They savor the act of courtship just like anyone else.

This was a moment that Billy Dee and Marlene had cultivated. All the cafeteria lunches, the movies, the little jokes, the strolls through the park and the city had created this moment that was full with a rich intensity. His cock was hard and she felt the tip of it against her belly. Her pussy was drenched and ready for him. He rolled on top of her. He continued to kiss her mouth and her face. As he looked into her eyes he whispered, "I want you so much," and smiled while his cock entered her slowly. The size was perfect and filled her nicely. She gasped and he pulled back and shoved it into her. He continued to wait a second and then shove it in. God, this was hot. No one had taken such control when fucking her. His Southern cool proved a heated powerhouse waiting to be released. The next shove she met him fuck for fuck. She was so wet and so juicy that they started slipping and sliding. He continued to rub his thumbs over her nipples while he was doing this. This sent an additional electrical charge to her clit.

She pushed him over so he was on his back. She sat on his cock and smiled as she reached for his hands so they could be joined while they made love. She pushed herself up and down on his cock and then sat on it and swirled her hips around to stimulate her clit. She was close to orgasm, but wanted to prolong it, so she hopped off and went down between his legs. She grabbed the base of his penis and held tight while she put it in her mouth. She tasted her own juices, which were sweet and tangy at the same time. She twisted her hand at the base of his cock while she sucked to her heart's content. She went up and down and followed with her hand. His cock was beautiful. It was deep brown and was accentuated by his tight black pubic hair. His balls were in a deep black sack that Marlene found very sexy, so sexy that she gave each ball a special slurpy suck into her mouth. He groaned to show he liked it. She smiled and slipped her finger into his anus. As she fingered his asshole, she sucked his balls and then moved on to deep-throating his cock. She gagged a bit because his cock was so damn big, not that she was complaining. She felt the thin skin tighten, so she continued her deep sucks while twisting her hand around the base. His hand grabbed her hair on the back of her head as he arched and grimaced. She tasted the saltiness of his cum as he came in spurts flowing down her throat. She swallowed it all.

Marlene kept her mouth on his cock until it started to deflate. She slowly removed her finger from his asshole and then climbed up to drape herself over his chest. He kissed her and said, "Thank you, that was wonderful," and smiled that beautiful smile into her face. "You're welcome," she said as she kissed his lips. They sighed into each other's bodies.

Marlene had had several men in her life over the years. She had worked hard to evolve as a spiritual human being and to be a loving partner who could be present in the moment. There were many times when she had been discouraged that people didn't match the image of them she had worked so hard to cultivate. Billy Dee met her expectations 100 percent. She was so grateful in that moment. She never could have dreamed that a man ten years younger could be such a fulfilling partner.

Cougars are known for their independence and personal freedom, but there are quite a few who actually fall in love and marry the young men they have become involved with. Demi Moore, Tina Turner, Susan Sarandon, and Geena Davis are a few of the women who have broken the taboo of older women dating younger men. And I say, "Good for them!"

THINGS YOU NEVER SAY TO A COUGAR

→ So, how old are you?

→ I wasn't born then.

→ That music is from the old days.

→ Don't you have an iPod?

→ You don't use Botox do you?

→ Do you dye your hair?

→ You might want to work out more to tighten things up.

→ Cosmopolitans are so old fashioned.

Let's Play Pool

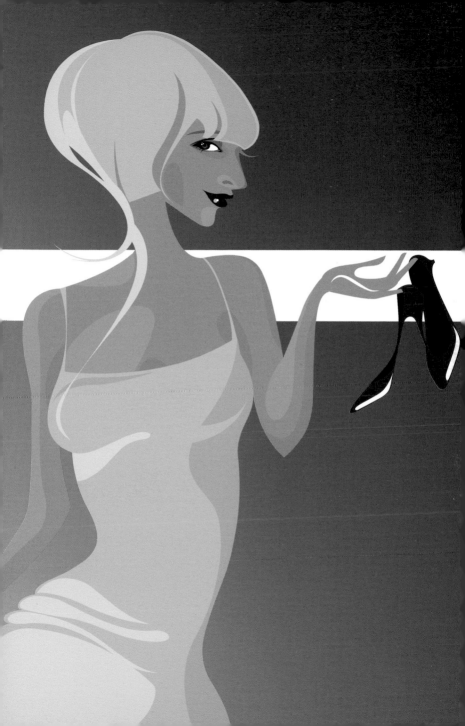

Every Saturday afternoon, my friend Myra takes a yoga class. Though she's almost sixty, she still has the metabolism to treat herself to a nice greasy hamburger afterward. Not to mention that she particularly liked the handsome young bartender, Jason, at the neighborhood pub.

Myra was recovering from a cheating husband. She'd recently started her own company and was gradually gaining confidence in herself. It showed in her body, and her mind wasn't bad, either. One particular day, she had a thought . . . about Jason.

Jason always greeted her with a big, "Hi, how are ya?" and poured her favorite beer. He was sweet and asked how her job was. This day was no different. He reminded her of a time in her life when things weren't so complicated. Jason had that Abercrombie & Fitch look—blond, blue eyes, and a strong looking chest. She noticed that his hair kind of fell over his right eye. She dreamily watched him and wondered what it would look like if she unbuttoned the top two buttons of his white shirt. She had the strongest urge just to put her nose against that skin and inhale deeply.

"Would you like another beer, Ms. Jacobs?"

"Uh, no. Tell me, what are you doing later on, Jason?"

"Well, I am working late here at the bar, ma'am."

"Like some company closing up?"

Why mince words? She liked what she saw and was going after it. Jason's eyes twinkled as he told her what time to come later on. She would definitely keep him company while he was closing.

Myra went home and contemplated her latest conquest. She had discovered she liked going after younger men. She didn't have time for men in their sixties. She found them too set in their ways and way too uptight. Young men could keep up with her and didn't mind if she took off afterward. They were just what the doctor ordered to give her a break from her high-powered life and mend her broken heart.

She walked into her dressing closet and dropped her yoga bag on the floor. With her hands on her hips, Myra contemplated what she wanted to wear for tonight's dalliance. She felt supersexy and decided to give this lad an experience to remember. She opened her lingerie drawer and ran her fingers over the finery. Mmmm, a black silky push-up bra, matching panties, and garter belt. Later that evening, she snapped the final garter in place with a pair of vintage black seamed hose. She slipped on a pair of Christian Loboutin black stilettos and nothing but a black trench coat.

A long leg snaked out of the cab as Myra walked out to the pub. She walked through the smoky bar past the pool table and sighted Jason wiping up the bar top. The place seemed to be emptying out. She watched and nearly swooned as his magnificent back stretched to lift a box. She realized it would be inappropriate to rip the shirt right off his back at that moment.

"Why don't you have a glass of wine while I finish up?" he said and placed a glass in front of her.

She crossed her legs and felt the silk against her bare thigh. The feel of it went straight to her pussy.

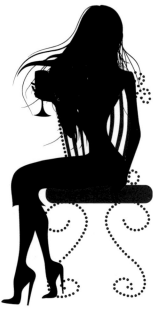

In a few minutes, he sat on the stool facing her. His legs fit nicely on either side of her kneecaps. She was still wearing her coat. Soon they were talking. Little electrical currents shot out each time their knees touched. There is something about that initial moment of making contact with a person that is so titillating. She noticed his fingertips, the length of his fingers, the sturdy boots he had on his feet, the gold chain around his neck with the little gold cross. It fit right at the base of his throat, which was a perfect place for a kiss. She thought it was so much fun to take someone in for the first time up close.

"Hello," he smiled. She noticed he had a rakish grin while his hair continued to fall over his eye. For some reason it tickled the inside of her stomach.

They chatted a bit about her yoga class. She listened to him tell stories about the drunks at the bar. He made her laugh with his funny descriptions. It felt good just to be silly, which was something she had lost with her husband.

"Do you know how to play pool?" he asked.

"No, why don't you show me?"

They strolled over to the table. The green felt looked intriguing. Jason took hold of a long pole and chalked the tip of it. The act was so suggestive she couldn't help but smile and look away. He set up a rack of balls on the table and then bent over to make his play. Myra was starting to spark at this point, and every move this young man made created more heat for the fire. His strong leg muscles curving over his butt were a sight to behold. She slowly walked behind him to the other side. Her stilettos clicked seductively on the floor. Well, she thought it was important to get a good look at the lay of the land.

"It's your turn," he said to her with his lips slightly parted.

"What do I do?" she asked as she grabbed the pool cue. He walked up to her and stood behind her with his arms around her. The warmth surrounding her body was thrilling. He placed his hands over hers on the pool cue. Hmmm.

A girl could get used to this, she thought. It would be easy to stay in this position all night.

"You hold the cue like this, and focus on the white ball and then hit it like this," he showed her.

Myra couldn't even hear what Jason was saying at this point. Her body had taken over and she was all physical sensation. She found young men did this to her. That was the fun of just letting herself feel and be open to her erotic sensations.

"Well, first you want to bend over like this," he said.

"Mmmm," she acknowledged. She noticed that her ass fit perfectly in his crotch. The heat that emanated from his body was enticing. He smelled of smoke and beer. She settled in closer and felt a bulge nudging her behind. She went back to noticing his hands as they guided her in using the cue. She imagined them touching her body.

"You want to do it like this," he stated.

"Oh, really?" she looked to her side into his face. She let her lips skim his cheek. The day-old whiskers prickled her lips. She noticed the bulge seemed to be growing.

"Yes, you do," he countered and threw the pool cue down on the table while he grabbed her waist. This was what she had in mind. She twisted her body to meet his and wrapped her arms around him as she felt hard muscles along his sides. Her breath escaped her at the feel of him. She noticed his lips were ample to the point of being edible. He took his time and slowly sought the inside of her mouth, feeling its smoothness. Myra thought, *This was definitely worth waiting for.*

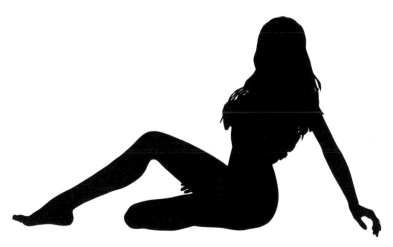

Enough with the subtle foreplay—they both dove in. It was hot and it was going to be dirty. They sought each other's mouths with a vicious hunger. She tore open his white button-down shirt and threw it on the floor. Then she pulled off his T-shirt. *Oh, sweet lord, his chest must have been chiseled in heaven.* Each pink nipple greeted her with attention.

Men have often been known for their lust for the visual, but women are capable of the same desire. Cougars particularly thrive on the visual heat that is stirred by looking at a body that scorches with its perfection. It can be marvelous to have the freedom of shamelessly going after a young man and tasting his fruits. Myra found it so freeing to let her passion run wild and not be restrained by social obligations.

Myra ran her fingers up along his chest. Her eyes just about rolled up and back into her head at the silky feel of it. The skin on his chest was smooth and taut, flawless. She wanted to just bite into him, so she took a nip out of his throat. He bucked in response. He took her waist and sat her on the edge of the pool table. Isn't this what pool tables were designed for? He took a moment to focus on her eyes and undo the belt to her trench coat. *Oh, yes, the trench coat.* She placed her hands behind her to brace herself for the show she was going to give him. Gradually he undid each button one by one. She ran the top of her leg between his legs.

Jason's eyes came alive when he uncovered her sexy costume. She enjoyed having the ability to allow her sensuality to ooze out. He stepped in between her legs and held her face while he kissed her. He left a trail of kisses down her throat and down to her breasts. She lay back as he continued kissing down her belly and caressed her hips. He pulled her panties down. She imagined how sweet her own perfume smelled. That was another bonus of being older—an appreciation of your own juices. He slowly licked her pussy's lips. Then he alternated between sucking her pearl and using his tongue to swirl around and around. He inserted one finger in her pussy to wet it and then gently slid it inside her anus. He went back to sucking.

Myra concentrated on the tongue massage. Jason had started off slowly, which she needed to let herself climb into it. She felt her clit and anus come to attention. The muscles inside her thighs began to tense up as she felt herself tightening them together. She felt a heat start to swell in her pelvis. He intensified his sucking as she felt herself start to release the flood of exhilaration pulsing through her cunt. "Aieeeee!"

she screamed as her thighs squeezed the sides of his face. Her back arched in response.

Jason stood up. His face was flushed and his cheeks were moist. He grabbed Myra's waist, pulled her up to her feet, and had her bend over the pool table. Myra was primed as he slid himself right in to home base. She had no inhibitions and welcomed him fully, moaning as his finger moved again into her ass. He loved this about her. She braced herself on the table. Her insides were blistering against the skin of his cock. It propelled him to thrust deeply. He held her hips and quenched his own need to possess her body at that moment. He took his cock out now and entered the tight cavity he had prepared with his fingers. He went slowly and then started to fuck her there once he felt she had relaxed enough for him to pulse more freely. He felt his own legs tighten and prepare for the tsunami. He screamed, "Oh fuck!" as he shot forth then. He fell over onto her back and just stayed there for a moment. Myra was warm and sweaty underneath him, in a daze.

They both sat on the edge of the pool table and let out a big breath trying to regain their composure. He was just as excited by her. "It was unbelievable to see this tall, luscious woman walk down the bar just for me," he told her. His hand roamed down the side of her leg, feeling the silky stocking. "You have the most amazing legs and you know just how to cross them—God, so slow, so sexy. I was trying not to stare at you so I didn't look like a fool." He snapped one of her garters. They took a moment to look at each other and burst out laughing. They fell back on the table and rolled onto each other and giggled senselessly. The bar was officially closed.

The Trainer

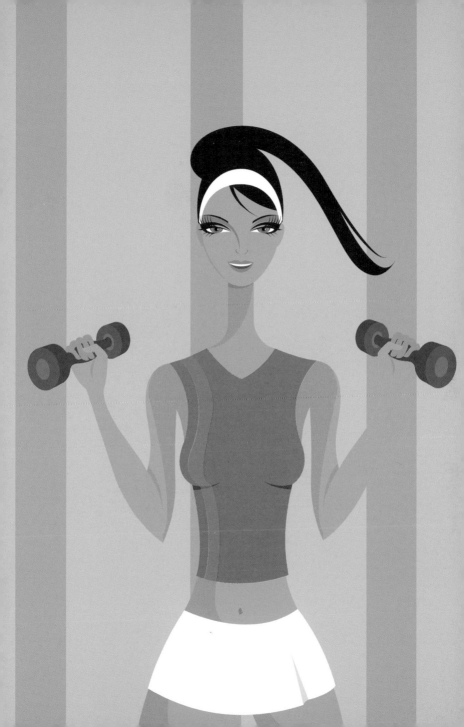

Lila was one of these brilliant women in her forties who had a difficult time getting past date number one. She had done therapy, AA, and every other self-help endeavor to try to correct any issues she may have had. She finally came to the conclusion that she was fine and she just needed to have a good time in life. She did the personals on Match.com and Nerve.com and even JDate. Dating had become a second job for her. She was very discouraged that so many men her own age only wanted to meet women who were much younger than them. It just didn't seem fair. *Well, fuck 'em,* she thought, *what is good for the goose is good for the gander.*

Lila worked out at Equinox, a chic health club in midtown Manhattan. She found it helped relieve the stress from work and dating, but it also helped her keep her figure. She was a classic cougar in that she kept herself in tip-top shape physically. As a result, she looked about ten years younger than she was. Lila had a personal trainer at the club. He must have been twenty-five at the most. He was 6'5", with strawberry-blond hair, and muscles that went on forever. She thought he would be perfect for one of those huge underwear ads in Times Square. The first day that Lila met him for a session, they hit it off right away.

He was laid back, but very funny. He asked her what she wanted to work on.

"Well," Lila said, "I want to work on my butt, legs, abs, stomach, and arms."

Lila thought to herself she would rather work on his butt, but that was another story.

"So basically you want a new body?"

"Uh, yeah, that about covers it."

They both had a good chuckle over that.

"Is there hope for me?" she asked.

"I don't think it is as bad as you think. Let's see what you've got." He started her off on the treadmill for twenty minutes. She was in pretty good shape, so this wasn't too bad. Then it was on to weight lifting. She followed him to the weight lifting area in the club. Jesus, she would follow him anywhere. He had her sit back to do some flies with fifteen-pound weights. He stood between her legs and guided her arms. She was wearing her best lululemon workout outfit, but was keenly aware of how close their barely clothed bodies were. He raised her hands so she was holding the weights above her breasts. Ay yi yi. There was something about this that was so intimate. His crotch was right at her eye level. Lila thought this was going to work out just fine.

Lila had a very busy schedule, so she inquired with the trainer if he did house calls and found out he did. *Oh goody!* They scheduled Tuesday and Thursday at 4:30 P.M. This way she could end her day with a bang and work out any tension she may have. Let's just say her intentions weren't that noble. She frequently worked out of her office at home and had a great open space in her loft.

The trainer arrived early the first Tuesday. Lila was already dressed in a black workout top with crisscrossing straps in back and matching pants that left little to the imagination. She worked hard to stay in shape and it showed. Like many cougars, she enjoyed feeling tight and firm. She was an empowered woman who enjoyed taking care of her body and relished the results she procured. This is a major characteristic of the cougar. Her body is fine-tuned and she delights in taking care of it and using it to its maximum for her sexual dalliances.

The trainer walked in the door. There was no doubt about it.

He was a large man. He had trained as a semipro baseball player, and sported a great pair of legs. Lila tilted her head and tried not to drool. Lila didn't mess around when it came to working out. Her space featured a bike, treadmill, weights, and plenty of mats for floorwork. She didn't mess around when it came to almost anything. She was ready for just about anything. The question was: Was he? He had her lie

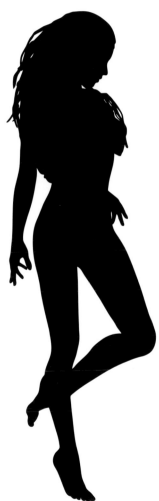

down on the floor while he sat next to her. He sat very close and kept his hand on her abdomen to help her catch her C curve while she did crunches. This was killing her, but it certainly was a sweet pain. He then knelt behind her and kept his hands underneath her shoulders. She would do anything this guy asked her to do. Her head was basically in his lap. He developed a routine for her that would tighten her already spectacular body. Each week he would take her through it and change it up a bit so she didn't get bored. *Fat chance.*

One day after a session they took a water break.

Lila was trying to rub out a knot in her shoulder. The trainer was watching her assiduously and offered, "I can get that out for you."

Lila raised an eyebrow and said, "Be my guest."

The heat of his fingers seeped into her sore muscles. Slowly he circled his thumbs into her deltoids. Lila closed her eyes, "Ah, yes, that's it. Right there."

"I can feel it. Just try to relax and breathe into it,"

God, this man can give a massage. There was nothing worse than a man with scrawny fingers who couldn't massage worth shit. His thumbs went down toward her lower back along her spine and over her kidneys. Her head kind of lolled back. Her breathing started to slow down. His thumbs continued their circular journey along her screaming muscles. He said, "Here, lie down so I can get to you better."

Lila thought, *I would love for you to get to me better.* She nestled her head to her side with an impish smile. He straddled her back, so it almost seemed as if he was sitting on top of her butt. Of course, in her mind, he could sit on top of her butt anytime. Now he started to cook. He used his whole body to work on her tired muscles. He swirled, he pushed, he prodded, and he smoothed her entire body. Lila was reduced to a groaning gob of goo.

He bent over with his hands on her shoulders and

asked, "How are you doing?"

With eyes closed, Lila murmered, "Just fabulous, mmmmm." At that very moment, the trainer brushed his lips across the back of her neck.

Lila felt like Sleeping Beauty coming out of a deep sleep as she turned around and slipped her arm around his neck to seek out more from those wonderful lips. Lila noticed his skin was luminous, guiding her forward. He had on a sleeveless T-shirt that did wonders for his chest. She swung one leg over his and let out a deep sigh. His arm slid down and grabbed her waist. To Lila, there was nothing like a man this size because she loved the sense of being enveloped by manliness. As much of a cougar and empowered woman as she was, there was nothing like this feeling. She felt it was embedded deep within her, and embraced it. As she consciously did this, their mouths and hips interlocked in synchronicity.

Just grabbing on to this all-American body was almost an extension of her workout. She was ready to take him on. *Hold on, baby, 'cause I'm coming,* she thought. He certainly was ready for the challenge. He grabbed her back and fixed her readily on his hip plexus. Here were two physical beings in their prime who were primed for each other.

There was a flurry of clothing as they stripped.

He grabbed her and had her hold on to the ledge of the windowsill. They were both naked and standing in front of the window. She presented her derriere and he entered her from behind. The lights weren't on, but the feeling of standing in front of the window for all to see had to be the most exhilarating experience she had ever had and she didn't care. She wanted to be there, she wanted to do this.

One thing about older women: they are full of juiciness. She totally opened her cunt to take him in.

"Fuck me, just fuck me," she growled. She bent her head to brace herself.

The trainer complied. His cock was nice and hard. She bucked her head and fucked him back. In return, he gave it right back to her. He started to move at a faster pace. He held on to her hips to guide himself deeper, then harder. She could take it hard, so he rammed it up her pussy. She needed it, she wanted it.

"Goddammit, just FUCK me," she ordered. Her hair flicked back as her head jerked to take in the cock of the century. Her breasts swayed with each violent thrust. My God, she was so alive, every nerve and muscle in her body was alive as if she were a vampire sucking the blood from a young man she had nabbed from the street. She didn't need to come, but she reached a point where she went on her tiptoes, held on to the window ledge and growled full blast. Her legs tensed and she went in for the royal fuck. *Whew.*

A woman at this age loves to be fucked, she needs it, she craves it, and she fully relishes it when she gets it. This is a major characteristic of a cougar. She savors a nice cock and a good fuck.

She took a deep sigh and let her head fall back as she started to slow down. The trainer came in close and wrapped his arms around her, holding each breast. They fell down on the settee and lay there for a minute in each other's arms, coming back down to earth.

Lila stated, "My God, darling, that was one hell of a workout. Do they show you that in Phys Ed?"

"Yes," he said, "It is called the 'fuck-the-pussy routine,' and it has marvelous effects every time."

They both grinned as they lay there.

She popped her head up, "Hey, are you hungry?"

"Yeah," he said.

"Let's go to the kitchen," she suggested with a devious grin.

THE TRAINER
AND THE BATH

Lila and the trainer padded down the hallway toward the kitchen. Lila popped into her bathroom and pulled out white terrycloth robes for each of them. Lila opened her large stainless steel fridge and they both stood in front perusing their choices.

Lila took the trainer's hand, where she led him to her luxurious bathroom. Her pad was so spectacular it had once been featured in *Home and Garden*. Her bathroom was her sanctuary, so she had wanted it designed with a Zen-like atmosphere. It was in soft greens with an Asian influence. She turned on the Jacuzzi, which could easily fit two people. She poured in some Jo Malone jasmine and peppermint bath soap and lit matching candles all over the room. She flicked a switch and some smooth jazz started to softly play. She looked at the trainer and stated, "Shall we?"

"Absolutely," he replied.

They both climbed into the tub. She turned it on to a slow bubble. They both sat back and let the warm water soothe their sexed-out bodies. Lila thought it felt very good on her pussy—very good on everything, for that matter. She lay back and looked at her blond god sitting opposite her. Man, he was fantastic. She took her red-toed foot and pushed her toes up and underneath his cock and balls. They felt soft and mushy on her toes, very nice, actually. She loved the way they fell over her foot. He smiled back at her and within a minute he started to respond and get hard.

He looked at her and invited, "Care to hop on?"

"Oh well, if I must."

She moved over to her knees and then her feet. She squatted right over that behemoth member of his. She was a bit sore, but this was no time for complaining. She placed her hands on either side of the Jacuzzi and slowly hoisted herself up and down, up and down. Lila thought there was nothing like fucking your brains out to utter satiation. This was not an easy position for anyone to maintain, no matter how good the cock was. She climbed off and slipped back. She grabbed a bottle of bath oil and poured it in her hand.

"I think we should make sure you are moisturized, darling. Don't you think?"

"I fully believe in moisturization."

She grabbed the base of his cock and rubbed the oil around on his penis. It was the perfect lubricant. She put her full body into the intimate massage,

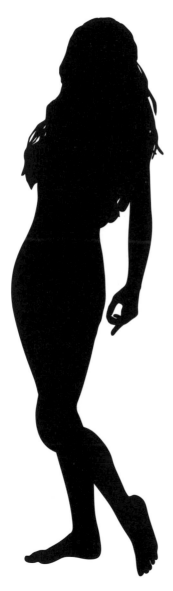

swirling and pulling, up and down, more and more. The soft candlelight flickered on the bubbling water foaming around their supple bodies. They could have made the cover of a hot romance novel. His cock responded by growing tauter and tauter. She liked what she saw. Lila found she was very much turned on by the visual presentation of a hot male body. The trainer fit the bill perfectly.

As she perused his body, she admired his pink nipples, his gleaming pecs, the bulging muscles in his arms, the thick neck, his wonderfully strong thighs. She had to admit this was better than bathing alone. She circled her finger around the rim of his cock and through his little crevice, taking time to scrape her fingernails underneath the shaft. She knew she was getting close to bringing him to climax as his face started to grimace. She increased the pressure and continued to twist her hand around him. Finally the moment arrived and she was thrilled to give it to him. She pumped him hard as his cum squirted up into the air and onto his chest in three hot squirts.

"And the judges give that a resounding ten," Lila proclaimed.

She reached over and grabbed a giant loofah sponge and soaked it with warm sudsy water. She proceeded to squeeze it all over his body several times as he lay back and literally soaked it in. The air was heavy with candlelight and the scent of jasmine and mint. They lay back, resting their heads on the edge of the Jacuzzi, and the tub bubbled on.

HOW TO ANSWER THE QUESTION, "SO HOW OLD ARE YOU?"

It's going to happen, so try not to freak out. I would address it before he asks or allude to it in a prior conversation—"Well, I am about twenty-five years older than you." If he asks you right after sex, tell him, "This isn't the best time to be asking me this, but I am fifty." Or "Let's discuss this later when I am not so vulnerable." But your best defense is to talk about it prior to sex or during your first date. Defense is your best offense.

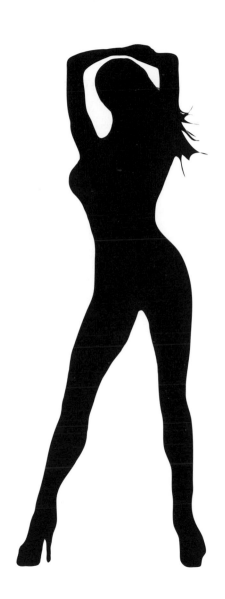

Career Girl Wins an Award

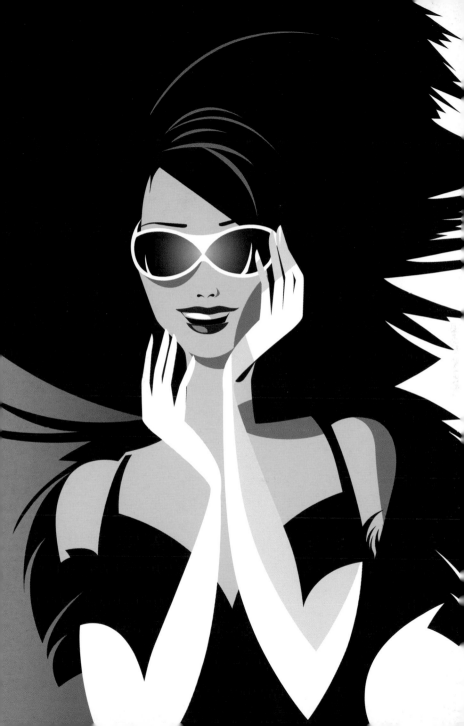

Melina was a petite gal from L.A. She was known for clicking down the street in her stiletto heels at an ungodly pace. She wore her dark hair shorn in a pixie-like do with a bright swash of MAC red lipstick. Melina was forty-one, which some considered the new thirty. If you took one look at her, you would have thought so.

Melina was all about her career. Her life wasn't about home-cooked meals and having children. It was about being top in her field and writing the screenplay that would get her the best damn picture that people would be talking about for years. Well, she had done it.

Melina definitely epitomized the new cougar. She didn't set out looking for a young man in particular. She actually met her boyfriend while at a pharmacy. She had been looking at cold medicines and was perplexed about what to choose. He happened to have been standing in the aisle; he offered her some help. Turns out he was a doctor, her very own McDreamy. He hadn't been too hard to miss. He was 6'3", with curly light brown hair and blue eyes. He had on a pair of jeans that showed off a muscular pair of legs. They had struck up a conversation and the rest was history. They had now been seeing each other for about a year. Since both worked so hard, they didn't see one another very often—and when they did, they didn't waste time. That was another bonus of being a cougar: being secure enough not to need the constant reassurance that her man is thinking of her. She can go straight to the bed, or table, or wherever she chooses to find her pleasure.

Melina enjoyed being erotically creative and found that a younger man had no problem with that. Frequently, older men got stuck in always having sex in the same position or fantasy, which was such a bore. Switching sex up and being open to whatever whimsy struck her fantasy was how Melina chose to go about her lovemaking. The doctor loved it. He found that younger women weren't as creative or free. He marveled at Melina's imagination and the delightfully devious ideas she came up with. He never knew when she would surprise him and that was exactly what kept him attracted to her.

Recently they went on a hike together. They were roaming around in the woods when they came across some very unusual mushrooms. Melina was on her knees looking at them when the doctor came over to look, too. She looked up at him with that gleam in her eyes. She slowly unzipped his shorts. The doctor smiled with delight.

"I think I am inspired," she said. She pulled out his cock. "Oh look, a giant mushroom! I think I'll eat it."

With that she promptly put it in her mouth. She began to suck on the knob of his well-proportioned cock.

"Mmmm," she said while the doctor closed his eyes and started to groan.

She sucked with vivacity. She traced the rim with her tongue and slid it into his little crevice. She went back to sucking. She held on to the base of it and started to twist her hand around it. She spit on it for good luck and better maneuverability. She grabbed underneath his balls and started to massage them. Then she pulled them down a bit as she deep-throated his cock. He was rock solid.

"I've never seen a mushroom do this before," she exclaimed.

"Oh fuck," he said and grabbed her from underneath her armpits and placed her back against a humongous tree.

"I need to fuck you—*now*."

He pulled down her khaki shorts in a second. Her pussy was well lubricated at this point. He shoved his cock in her immediately. She bent her knees a little and braced herself against the rough bark.

"Ouch!"

"Shut up and take it."

She smiled and loved it. "Then fuck me hard," she ordered.

And fuck he did. His cock was thick and a good six and a half inches. Melina loved him ramming that thing in her cunt. It was so wild to be outside—what if someone came along the path? It made it even sweeter. The doctor pumped like a wild animal and bit her neck as he started to come. She tipped her pelvis forward and took all of his cum.

"There's your fuck," he said.

"I never knew mushrooms could be so much fun," she said with a smile.

When the day came that Melina received her nomination for best screenplay, she knew exactly who she was asking to go with her: the doctor, her favorite piece of arm candy. He was certainly more to her than that, but he sure would look hot in a tuxedo on that red carpet. Yum.

Preparing for the awards was part of the trip. She found herself in the delightful position of having designers send her gowns to her home in Malibu. She decided on a classic black, slinky number by Chanel. This would elongate her petite figure and dark hair. She chose a diamond necklace by Harry Winston complemented by a little diamond star in her hair. The doctor had chosen a classic tuxedo by Giorgio Armani.

The day arrived. Melina found herself a bit nervous not only about the chance of receiving a major award but also being escorted with a younger man. Would her peers make fun of her? Would they think she was cool for doing it? Would they talk behind her back? Well, Susan Sarandon had done it and so had Demi Moore, so why couldn't she? Dating a younger man so openly was new to her and it was still new to the world. Women were just starting to be open about their desires and flaunting it.

Well, she thought, *so will I.*

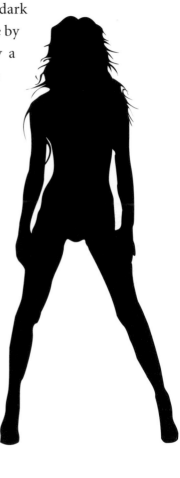

The door to the limousine opened. She looked at the doctor as he smiled and took her arm. She was really going to do this.

As she stepped out, she thought, *Here I am, world—cougarlicious. Eat your hearts out!*

The Designer

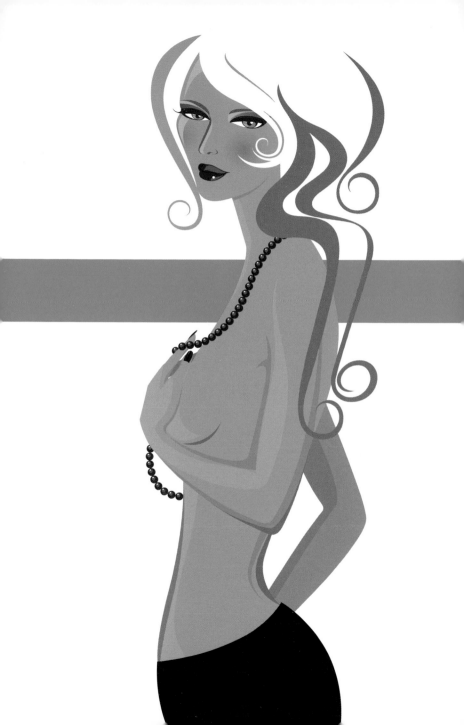

Georgia is a fifty-year-old photographer for *National Geographic.* When her husband of twenty years died unexpectedly from cancer, she dove into her work to keep her sanity. She traveled incessantly for the next five years.

Georgia was finally starting to be able to slow down and take a break and come to terms with the tragedy she had been dealt. She realized she was ready to start her life anew. She decided to start by updating her living space. She had bought the place with her husband, and she needed to change it up a bit, make it her own. A friend recommended a designer and she made an appointment. No time like the present.

The day of her appointment she got up like any other day, put on a pair of jeans and a T-shirt. She had lost weight since losing her husband. She loved to run when she was in foreign countries. It was a great way to see the land. She had recently grown out her hair and gotten it highlighted. Her makeup was as natural as possible, though she'd discovered sheer lip-gloss that promised to plump her lips.

Every morning Georgia went into town to her local coffee shop for a special java. That morning Georgia grabbed a paper and scone and sat down to enjoy the sunny morning. She noticed a stunning man walk in the shop. He was dressed right out of *GQ* with a creamy T-shirt, a wool cap, and incredible checked pants. It had been a long time since a man had caught her eye. This man was like a stallion. She noticed his back, wide and toned from serious weight lifting. She was truly in awe of this man's body. He was huge, maybe 6'8". Everything about him was rock solid. His legs were so long they were amazing. And his rear end was a force to be reckoned with—to her shock, she wanted to bite it. Wow, it had been a long time since she felt this way. It felt good to be alive again. She admired the view while she sipped her coffee.

Back at home, she waited for the designer. The doorbell rang at the appointed time. When Georgia opened the door, there was the young man from the coffee shop. She tried not to let her jaw drop on the floor.

"Uh, hi," she managed to eke out.

"Hi, I'm the designer," he said.

Georgia thought she was going to faint. Finally, she got her voice back.

"Come in, come in," she said. "This is my space."

She walked him in and couldn't believe this gorgeous creature was in her home. Her home was huge. It had exposed brick with beams and old wooden floors that had been buffed. It was easily large enough to allow for roller-skating. There was an area for shooting photos, a living room, and a dining area. The kitchen area was massive. Huge windows opened out onto the yard.

The designer walked around and took time to look at some of her photography on the walls and made a few measurements while he was at it.

"Let's sit down and chat a bit. I need to get a sense of who you are and what you are hoping to do in redesigning this space," he said.

What started out as a chat turned into a two-hour talk. This young man was innovative and confident in a very relaxed manner. He had a mischievous side that made her laugh. She wasn't sure, but thought maybe he was flirting with her. She couldn't help but notice his strong thighs as the material of his pants stretched over them. *Ay caramba*, this man was hot.

They chatted about all kinds of things. She asked him how he started his business and landed in Manhattan. She talked about her husband and her desire to change her space for her new life. He asked about her travels and inquired as to what had inspired her that they could incorporate into the space. Georgia loved this idea. She loved the rich colors of India and of the Orient. He got her to thinking about some interesting ideas that she found exciting. She ended up putting on one of her saris to show him the colors that she absolutely loved. As she twirled around, she hoped his mind might create some wonderful images not all about interior design.

The next day the designer called Georgia and asked if she could meet for lunch. He suggested a

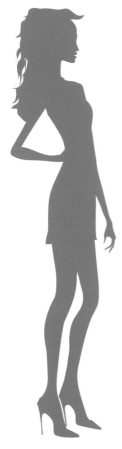

great restaurant around the corner from her, which featured the sort of architectural design that he thought she might like to see. Naturally, she accepted.

The next day, Georgia took extra care putting on her makeup. She fretted a bit about which pair of jeans to wear.

Then she thought, *What the hell am I doing? This guy is a kid and my designer—it isn't a date.*

She tugged on a fantastic pair of boots. She grabbed her pocketbook and keys, and right before she walked out the door she checked out her derriere in the mirror.

"I still got it," she said with a flick of her hair, and out she went. Her heels clicked as she strutted down the sidewalk. Georgia thought it felt good to be vital again. What the hell? She walked in the door of the restaurant and there he was.

Again, she found herself aroused by his looks. Georgia snorted and thought that drooling and panting were not exactly good ideas right at this moment. She would need to try to be somewhat calm and collected despite the fact that that her internal temperature appeared to be around 500 degrees.

"Hi," she said, and slipped into a chair of Marrakech design. She noticed the Byzantine chairs and woodwork. Each doorway was carved and rounded. The fabrics were in rich reds, greens, and golds. She loved it.

The waiter brought out what looked like a large spongy pancake and put it on the little round table in front of them. He then plopped little mounds of food around the edges of it. The aim was to rip pieces with the food on it. The designer ordered a bottle of wine to go with their meal. They both agreed that the food was actually Ethiopian, but who cared? It was marvelous.

The designer pointed out a few things in the restaurant that he thought they should consider, particularly the color design. He showed her the ideas he had sketched out and a few color swatches.

She loved all of it, and found herself getting quite enthused. It might have been the wine, it might have been the swatches, or it just may have been him.

A few days later, the designer stopped by to go over paint and fabric samples with her. He had chosen a very exotic combination of deep purples, reds, and gold. Georgia loved it. She also loved having him come over to her space. He just seemed to brighten up her day. While they were in the middle of throwing swatches all over the floor, the designer asked what she was doing over the weekend. Georgia kind of shook her head in disbelief. She didn't just hear what she thought she heard—did she?

"Well, I—um—am just hanging out," she said.

"Take a ride with me to the shore. I have a craving for a big gooey hot dog with all the fixings. It will be fun. What do you say?" he asked.

Georgia laughed. He was so unexpected, and it sounded like so much fun. It was wonderful to be old enough not to play games. She had nothing to lose!

She blurted out, "Oh, that sounds like a blast, let's do it."

"I'll pick you up Sunday around 10 A.M.," he promised.

Sunday, Georgia's buzzer rang. She grabbed her bag and raced down the stairs, leaving any caution behind. She figured that after all she had been through with the death of her husband, she needed to have some fun. Here was this fabulous young man offering it to her. She was ready for the adventure to begin. When she stepped outside on the sidewalk, there was the designer in a vintage mint-green Pontiac. She laughed and clapped her hands at the giant monstrosity waiting for her.

Oh, what fun, she thought.

The designer greeted her with a giant grin and threw open the door for her. She threw her bag in the backseat and sat on the front, which was the size of her sofa at home.

"Are you ready?" he asked.

"Oh, yeah, so ready. Let's go!" she exclaimed.

It was a glorious day. The sun was beaming and the air was perfectly delightful. Everything was starting to bloom and gave off a distinct smell of spring. They sped down the highway with the windows wide open and music blasting on the radio. When they arrived at the beach, they took a long walk along the boardwalk with the elderly couples and the young teens. They found their way to the hot dog stand. Georgia loved hot dogs and wondered how the hell he knew this. She ordered a dog with chili, onions, and cheese. My God it was good—nice and messy, just the way she liked it. Afterward, the designer held her arm as they walked down the boardwalk. It felt like a natural thing to do. They drove back sated and happy from such a fun day.

"Thank you so much. I had such a good time." Georgia said.

"Me, too. I'm glad you decided to come," he said and leaned over and gave her the sweetest kiss.

Wow, is this really happening? Georgia furrowed her brows in question. The designer had blindsided her. She wasn't expecting this at all and certainly wasn't looking for a hot stud. What would her husband have said about this? She decided he probably would encourage her to enjoy herself. It was a first date, though, and she went inside alone.

Later that night she was lying on her bed with her two cats. She couldn't help but think of the designer—those firm legs, that great back. She thought about running her hands slowly over every bit of him. Her mind wondered about what his body must be like without clothes. Since every bit of him was so large it stood to reason that his manhood must be. She let her hand wander down between her legs as she thought about it. She found that wondrous little nub and started to rub her middle finger in a circle over it. She thought about him getting hard underneath his pants, about rubbing her hand over it to make it even harder and making him crazy with desire. Finding his zipper on those jeans and unzipping them to have it jump out and greet her. It is hard and a deep pink and his pubic hair is light brown.

She imagined putting her face next to it. He might smell of musk, the woods, and soap. In her fantasy, she slips her hands underneath his ample balls. She puts each one in her mouth gently sucking. He groans in delight. *Suck, suck, slurp. Suck, suck, slurp.* She can't fit his whole cock in her mouth, so she uses her hand to help with her enticement. It is rigid. She knows she is bringing him to new heights when he grabs her shoulder hard. His eyes squeeze shut as she sucks him as deeply as she can without gagging. She pulls underneath his balls as she sucks with all her might. She feels the tight skin pulsing in her mouth pushing to release . . . and there it is.

Georgia moved her hand back to her chest. She opened her eyes to see her cat with his leg stuck in the air and his ears pushed back. He had a crazy look in his eyes and was looking at her as if to say, "What the hell do you think you are doing?"

"Mummy is having an orgasm, darling," Georgia laughed out loud.

The next day the designer called Georgia to ask if she could meet him at a store called Marrakech Imports.

Georgia gave an enthusiastic "Yes."

The store is in a huge building that used to house a cookie factory years ago. Georgia was stunned by the café and the shops, housed in rooms that still have some of the remnants from the cookie factory. There were unusual chairs and benches sculpted out of stone. The designer led her to a little shop that featured items from Marrakech. Georgia fell in love with it immediately. There was a stunning collection of colored ceramic tiles. The designer put his hand on her back as he showed her the collection. The heat

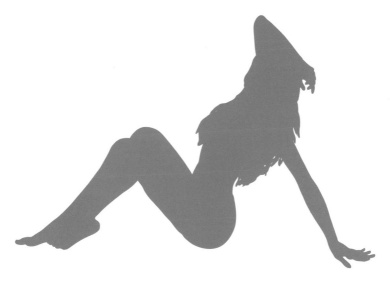

emanating from his hand made it very hard for her to concentrate. They picked some very cool stuff for the walls and floor in her kitchen area. She chose deep purple and red glass sconces to hang from the ceiling. The pièce de résistance was a leather footrest in the shape of a silver ball. It was just hilarious.

"Do you love it?" the designer asked and gave her a big smack of a kiss.

Georgia thought, *That isn't all I love.*

That week, things started to arrive at Georgia's loft and the designer started to redecorate. Georgia was starting to feel like she had been transported to the Middle East by the end of it. She luxuriated in the rich colors, beautiful glass, Byzantine furniture, and tiled floor. It was fabulous, and succeeded in doing just what she had hoped to do, which was to lift her mood and reawaken her inner spirit. She was alive and happy, thanks to the designer. As she stood admiring everything, the designer asked if she would like to go out for dinner and celebrate.

"That sounds terrific," she said.

That day Georgia went to her hair salon. She had her hair trimmed, highlighted, and blown out. She had a manicure and pedicure in fire-engine red. She felt like Dorothy in *The Wizard of Oz* with a "buff buff here and a buff buff there." She stopped at a shop down the street and picked up a chic little dress to show off her legs. This was fun, and what was even better, she was alive once again.

The designer rang her bell at the appointed time that night. Georgia walked out and was greeted by this stunning man, with his Pontiac, wearing a gorgeous pair of black pants and suede shoes. If there was anything that drove Georgia wild, it was a man wearing sleek suede shoes. It was a little fetish of hers and there was nothing she could do about it. What was even more incredible about him was that his clothes perfectly fit the lines of his amazing body—a pull here, a seam there, tight fabric everywhere. *Whew.* She was getting very warm.

The restaurant was lovely. It was new, so Georgia had never been there before. They drank white wine and Georgia tried wild striped bass with Fuji shrimp. The pairing of sauces, spices, and accoutrements was enough to send her tongue into orbit. As they ate, Georgia couldn't help but admire the fine line of the designer's jaw. He had such a strong face, which fit his masterful body. She noticed his eyes were a deep sea green. His hands were strong with long fingers and calluses that felt somewhat rough as he held her hand.

His eyes twinkled and he traced his finger in and out of hers. She wasn't sure she could make it through dinner without crawling over the table and attacking him right there in public.

"Let's get the check, shall we?" he asked.

"Absolutely," she responded.

"Would you like to see my place?"

"Yes."

This was the moment she had been anticipating. Every cougar is in tune to anticipating this moment. The designer lived on the other side of town. She knew his place would be fabulous, but wasn't fully prepared even so. Let's just say it was total sumptuousity. There were big comfortable chairs, and a giant Buddha greeted them, seeming to wink hello. A chubby calico cat came running out to greet his master. The designer picked him up and gave him a big kiss. "This is Max."

He poured two glasses of champagne and grabbed her hand.

"I have something I want to show you."

They walked out to the backyard. There were several cozy lounge chairs with end tables and a Zenlike fountain and bamboo trees. *Bamboo trees?*

"I am so glad I met you, Georgia. Here is to your new life. I hope I am a part of it."

Georgia felt a bit weak in the knees. He wrapped his arm around hers so they could drink from their glasses. It was heavenly. He put his glass down and then hers. She thought, *This is it. This is the moment.*

He wrapped his arm around her waist and leaned down to kiss her. It was rare that a man was so tall he had to lean toward her, and she loved it. His lips were soft but strong. His arms were solid under her hands. My God, he was remarkable. His tongue searched her mouth slowly at first as if to gently seek out the territory. She welcomed him and greeted him with hers. Even his tongue matched the rest of his body: it was strong, soft, and smooth all at the same time.

At that moment, he grabbed her body and pulled it to his with full strength. It was as if a switch went off inside him. A grunt of sorts came out of him and it went straight to Georgia's cunt. This is the kind of thing most women lust after in the bedroom—a man taking control with full force and showing his passion and strength.

This man certainly had strength, and the passion was intense. She wrapped her leg around his. He grabbed her even harder, so she was leaning backward as if they were performing a tango. He lifted her up and onto one of the lounge chairs nearby. It was big enough for both of them. She was on her back as he placed himself on top of her. The full force of this

She lost herself in his groin. She smelled it, she licked it, and just plain rubbed her face in it. Then she took her head and draped her hair up and down his body. She could tell he really liked this. She felt inspired.

The designer grabbed her and spun her over. He bent down on his hands and knees above her and pulled her panties off with his teeth.

Oh yeah, she thought, *Oh yeah.*

She was drenched. He went down between her legs and took one long lick with his enormous tongue and then gave her the tongue-lashing of her life. He then took two of his long fingers and pushed them inside her. Georgia thought, *There is nothing better than having someone lick you and use their very nimble fingers.* (With which sentiment, dear readers, I have to agree.)

She brought her hips to his lips and raised her arms behind her head. She felt totally open. She closed her eyes as she felt the sensations come alive. There was that familiar tingle. She could feel it building. He kept going at it. *Oh, fuck, this was good.* It was as if a current was circling the area where his tongue was and her heat emanating. She was a volcano ready to flow. There it was, she felt it coming and yes, there it was. She erupted and growled all at once.

"Just do me!" she screamed.

He wasn't waiting to be told. This man intuitively knew what to do. He was on his knees getting ready. He plunged into her full throttle.

"This is your cock, now fuck me," he said as he grabbed her hips.

Georgia was in fuck heaven. His rigid shaft was perfect. Something in her kicked in and she started bucking as if she were a wild bronco. She was in a frenzy and he was right there with her. He took his cue and plunged right back into her. She continued her equestrian dance and bucked with abandon. *Sweet mother, this was almost worth waiting five years for.*

Then she could feel the designer tense up, which told her he was about to come.

"Give it to me," she said, "just give it to me."

And give it to her he did.

Later they went downstairs and put on some cashmere robes. They were snuggled in front of the fireplace on the big cushy sofa with a lovely bottle of wine. Max, the cat, had decided to join them.

The designer reflected on his first meeting of Georgia. "You know, when I first met you, I was blown away with how gorgeous you are. And your body, God, it is so womanly, just lovely. And when you put on that sari, I thought I would die. I just about fell in love right then and there. And your photography,

McBride, Susan. *The Cougar Club: A Novel*. Avon, 2010. Print.

When three best friends reawaken and agree to turn their lives into sexual escapades, a fun fantasy ensues as these three cougars hunt down their hot cubs.

Mulvey, Kate. *How to Date a Younger Man: The Cougar's Guide to Cubhunting*. London: Carlton, 2011. Print.

In her humorous text, Mulvey teaches a cougar everything she needs to know in order to be the successful, bold predator she really is.

Pre, Jolie du. *The Cougar Book*. Logical-Lust Publications, 2010. Print.

Edited by Jolie du Pre, these twenty-three stories written by some of the scene's hottest cougars and cubs are sure to have any interested reader indulging in the world of erotica.

Targosz, Cyndi. *Dating the Younger Man: A Complete Guide to Every Woman's Sweetest Indulgence.* Avon, MA: Adams Media, 2008. Print.

As an actress and model, Cyndi Targosz knows as well as anyone that women in the modern world are becoming more powerful than ever. Infused with real-life stories, Targosz speaks of using that power to go after those handsome, seemingly unattainable younger men.

DATING SITES FOR COUGARS AND CUBS

Meet local cubs and cougars alike at these top-ranked cougar dating sites:

www.icougardating.com
www.cougarinternational.ning.com
www.meetlocalcougars.com
www.cougarfling.com
www.cougarwomendating.net
www.vipcougarclub.com
www.clubcougar.us/what.htm
www.cougarhunter.ca
www.dateacougar.com
www.dateacougar.com/singles/newyork-cougar
www.cougared.com
www.urbancougar.com
www.cougarpatrol.com
www.cougardatingfree.com

COUGAR DENS

5150 Bar
15455 Valley Blvd
City of Industry, CA 91746

Balboa Cafe
3199 Filmore Street
San Francisco, CA 94123

Drink
348 Congress St
Boston, MA 02228

Elways
2500 East 1st St
Denver, CO 80206

Firefly on Paradise
3900 Paradise Rd
Las Vegas, NV 89109

Jim Porter's Good Time Emporium
2345 Lexington Rd.
Louisville, KY 40206

Liberatores
9515 Deereco Rd
Timonium, MD 21903

Local 16
1602 U St NW
Washington, DC 20009

Mecca Supper Club
6666 N. Northwest Highway
Chicago, IL 60631

Poseidon
1670 Coast Blvd
Del Mar, CA 92014

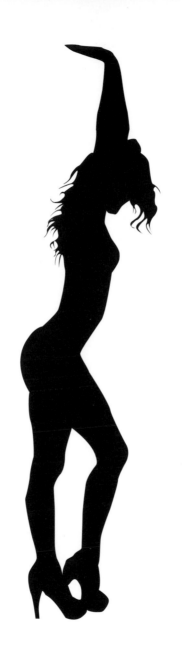

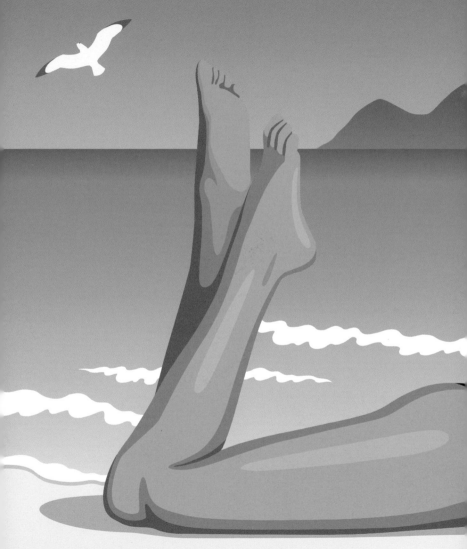

My Cougar Journal

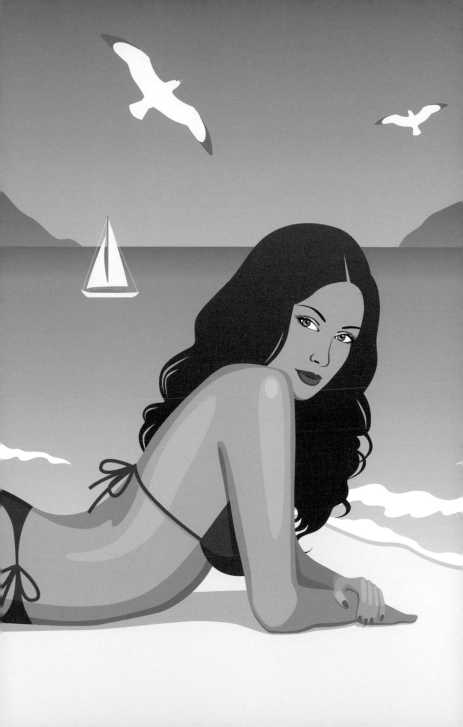

_____

_____

_____

_____

_____

_____

_____

_____

_____

_____

_____

_____

_____

_____

_____

_____

_____

_____

_____

_____

_____

_____

_____

_____

_____

_____

_____

_____

_____

_____